The Good News

You don't have to be a "sex goddess" to enjoy fantastic sex...but knowing how to cultivate your capacity for greater enjoyment in the bedroom may make you *feel* like one.

Better News

Just about any woman can become orgasmic by becoming more knowledgeable about how her body and mind work.

The Best News

Once a woman is able to achieve at least one orgasm, she can learn to respond—over and over and over again!

HOW TO HAVE MULTIPLE ORGASMS

JANALEE BECK

AVON BOOKS ◆ NEW YORK

Neither the author nor Avon Books recommend the use of illicit drugs. All matters regarding your health require a doctor's medical supervision.

The author wishes to express grateful acknowledgment to Michael Brooks, author of *Instant Rapport*, and Anthony Robbins, author of *Unlimited Power*.

AVON BOOKS
A division of
The Hearst Corporation
1350 Avenue of the Americas
New York, New York 10019

Copyright © 1993 by Janet Lee Becker
Published by arrangement with the author
Library of Congress Catalog Card Number: 92-90420
ISBN: 0-380-76938-7

First Avon Books Printing: February 1993

AVON TRADEMARK REG. U.S. PAT. OFF. AND IN OTHER COUNTRIES, MARCA REGISTRADA, HECHO EN U.S.A.

Printed in the U.S.A.

RA 10 9 8 7 6 5 4 3 2 1

Special Thanks to . . .

. . . My mother, who prefers to remain anonymous, for role-modeling unconditional love and for telling me about those mating butterflies.

. . . Susan, my twin sister, whose contributions of encouragement, seasoned expertise, and unfailing support I could not have lived without.

. . . David and Spomenka, my brother and sister-in-law, for their special commitment to keeping the spark alive in their rare relationship.

. . . Terry, my first love, for showing me the splendor of my sexuality.

. . . RDS, surprisingly, for unleashing the passionate Goddess within.

. . . My poker buddies for their appalling lack of knowledge about women's needs, thus serving as motivation to write this book.

Contents

Introduction:

Personal Notes to the Reader

I want to share some of the strange things that have happened to me since the original edition of my book came out over a year ago. The reactions of both men and women have been extremely interesting. Men either clam up or they ask a billion questions. Some spray their freshly squeezed orange juice all over me when I mention the title of my book. After apologizing, they share personal experiences ...like how heroic it feels to be with a multiorgasmic female...or how disheartening it feels to live with a sexually detached woman for twenty years.

Still others deny the existence of multiple orgasms altogether, and accuse me of lying; "You don't even know what an orgasm is," snapped a poker player in one of the largest card rooms in northern California. Instead of getting defensive, I merely stated that "an orgasm is an automatic reflex caused by stimulation to the clitoris that expresses itself in vaginal contractions, which last eight-tenths of a second each."

"Lucky guess," said one fellow, who then proceeded to support my contentions throughout the ensuing thirty-minute debate. Men, as much as women, need education in this area. Select gentlemen *know* that multiple orgasms exist because they've been on the welcoming end.

Women's reactions to the book, on the other hand, are much harder to predict. They typically fall into one of four categories:

I) Eager. Want to read it. Enthusiastic about the subject. Buy the book on the spot. (Approximately 20 percent.)

II) Curious. Want to talk about experiences—good and not so good. But prefer to read the actual book in private. (Approximately 45 percent.)

III) Uninterested. Don't want it. Beyond needing a book about sex, so they say. (Approximately 25 percent.)

IV) Offended. Actually say something negative or act in a defensive manner. (Approximately 10 percent.)

In my opinion, the women in groups III and IV need to read the book the most. I get the impression that they're close-minded about everything in their lives, including sexual exploration with a partner they love.

Unfathomable Connection

At a small get-together, I met a woman who had heard about my book through a friend. She came up to me and said, "I understand you've written seven steps to having better orgasms."

"Sort of," I answered. "I came up with the number after I analyzed what worked for me."

"Do you know what the first step should be?"

"What?"

"A trip to the shopping mall!" she exclaimed.

How strange that a woman connects shopping with sex at all! Does shopping make her feel more romantic after she's bought something or only when her husband buys it? I wonder if that's the way she feels good about herself. In either case, I think it's a sad statement.

Down-To-Earth Advice

I tell people that I'm an educator, not a clinical psychologist or a sex therapist; still many women approach me with personal information and so-called secrets. One woman brought me into her office, shut the door, and proceeded to tell me that she had been married for five years, yet never had a penetration orgasm.

"We're very much in love," she began. "My husband and I started reading your book together. I can have orally stimulated orgasms, but not the vaginal kind. What should I do?" she asked, leaning forward in her chair.

"Finish reading the book, practice those Kegel exercises, and keep trying" was all I could say on short notice.

Unhappily, I don't have the answers for everyone; but I do have practical, immediately useful suggestions for those interested in discovering heightened sexual pleasure. This woman, by the way, was a tall, leggy blonde who looked more like the author of the book than I do. Not that I'll crack a mirror, but I'm more the all-American girl-next-door type. Definitely not *Cosmopolitan* material. You'll usually find me in jeans; and, unless I'm going out, I hardly wear any makeup.

I do get my hair cut on a regular basis. When my hairdresser first saw my book, she said, "You look too sweet to have written a book like this." A second lady chimed in, "Yeah, you don't look the type."

I was struck by their comments. "I'm a healthy female . . . What else do I need as a qualification for enjoying sex?" I asked a little defensively. Apparently some women are just as guilty as men when it comes to stereotyping. *[Stereotype A: If you don't look sleazy, you must not be good in bed (or) Nice girls don't crave sex!]*

Mission Clarification

At that moment, my mission became clear to me. I want to go public to dispel myths. I envision myself on national television saying, "Yes, America, I wrote this book. As you can see, I'm not a sex goddess. But after a night of passion, I think, 'Sex doesn't get any better than this.' Isn't that what everyone should think about their love life?"

A week later, my book prompted a few females to discuss multiple orgasms at the health club. Another woman appeared from nowhere and, not realizing I was the author of the book, said, "I bet that woman doesn't do dishes!"

How bizarre, I thought. With my mission fresh in mind, I decided to enlighten her.

"Just because I enjoy my sexuality doesn't mean I don't do housework," I explained slowly. "Besides, with two preschoolers at home, I clean up so many messes, I wish I had stock in paper towels. Believe me, I do plenty of dishes."

These incidents, and more like them, made me realize that stereotypes are meaningless when it comes to any particular individual. *[Stereotype B: A multiorgasmic woman doesn't do anything ordinary in life (or) She must be a nymphomaniac!]* Think of all the stereotypes we carry around. Think of all the tall, dark, handsome guys you've met who were too shallow and conceited to be fun or sexy. I learned a long time ago that you can't judge a book by its cover. (And neither should you when it comes to men—or even when it comes to this book!)

The most wonderful men in the world aren't necessarily the most handsome. They're the ones who love us for who we are; the ones who treat us how they would like to be treated; the ones who accept the ups and downs of life; the ones who make us feel special in and out of the bedroom.

Only you can decide what you want in a man.

Maybe you already have him. Terrific. If not, go out and find what you want. Remember, don't exclude yourself from the club of sexually satisfied women just because you don't have the alleged appearance of a "sex goddess." All it takes is confidence in yourself and your mate.

Enjoying sex is a mind-set. So set your mind at ease and then practice, practice, practice!

1

If I Can Do It, So Can You

I've always wondered why women keep good secrets to themselves. I've discovered a great one—the secret of being multiorgasmic—and, personally, I want to share the mystery. I'm not writing this to impress you or make you jealous; I believe I have a mission to teach others how to heighten sexual pleasure. I also want to dispel myths and misconceptions about sexuality and help women reach their potential for female fireworks.

Since I just happen to be one of those women who climax easily, curious friends would ask me how I did it. At first, it was hard to explain. Through the years, though, I've found ways to reveal this knowledge. If I can help a handful of women brave the incredible sensation of multiple orgasms, then this book will have been worth the effort.

At the risk of sounding like a braggart, I want to tell you something: I've had more orgasms in seven days than most men do in seven months! I've never actually counted them one by one because that would take away from the experience. Why ruin a good thing, right?

My partner claims he can't figure it either—says he's too moved by the occasion. Without telling me, though, he counted them one time during a romantic minivacation and exclaimed, "Don't ever quote me . . . but now that I've experienced you, I think men got cheated!"

Must a Woman Be Multiorgasmic to Feel Fulfilled?

Not necessarily. It depends on the woman. One intense orgasm is perfectly satisfying for many women. In fact, this book stresses quality over quantity; but if a woman wants more,

I'm here to let her know it's possible...and very real. Men need this information, too. After reading my book to his wife, one thoughtful midwesterner said, "Honey, I'm sorry...I've been cheating you all these years ...I didn't know it could be like that for a woman. Tonight's going to be the best ever!" By the way, his wife thanked me profusely the next day.

While it's possible to have two, three, five, or more penetration orgasms in a single love-making session, discussing exact numbers misses the whole point. Goal setting is a marvelous idea for other activities in your life; it's just not appropriate in the bedroom. Put aside any goal you might have. Thinking you must have one, two, three, or more is the surest way to mechanical sex. How does one go about counting them anyway? As a close friend of mine told me, "I feel like the whole experience is one long orgasm." Approach sex with a fresh mind and a compassionate heart, not with numbers or time limits.

Most assuredly, it's not healthy to put up anyone's sex life as a touchstone from which to measure another. As sure as I live and breathe, someone would say my sexual experiences (or yours) lack variety, frequency, intensity, or creativity. There's one in every crowd eager to rain on someone else's parade. Ignore it.

Besides, swinging from a basket during sex may have been their idea of a good time, but it certainly is not mine. What's important is what goes on between two caring individuals, how compatible and ardent they are, how meaningful the relationship is, and so forth. I think men and women should willingly share ideas about sexuality without feeling threatened or judged.

If what works for me helps someone else enjoy sex a little bit more, great. If you believe *spirited sex* is important to your well-being, why not try to enhance it? Why not feed the libido and foster what you expect to do on a regular basis? Why not grow together as a couple in this area and discover lifelong pleasure? If reading this improves even one thing in the bedroom, so much the better.

My Philosophy on Good Sex

Did you know that you can actually cultivate a capacity to have orgasms? It takes practice and patience. Experts aren't sure what leads women to develop this aptitude, but I have my own philosophy. The essence of this book revolves around my beliefs that a woman must:

1) take chief responsibility for her own orgasm
2) internalize the belief that *spirited sex* is 90 percent mental
3) be in tune with her physical self

1) My philosophy about sex parallels my philosophy about life. Just as I believe each person is responsible for his or her own actions, I believe everyone is responsible for achieving his or her own orgasm. I call it *sex-equity lovemaking*. What I mean is that you need to rely primarily on yourself, not on your partner, to get what you want out of sex. First of all, you have to select a compatible mate. Lovers should also learn how to communicate their needs, verbally and otherwise, and know how their bodies respond to various stimulation. Women shouldn't expect their partners to read their minds or do everything—from foreplay to afterglow—perfectly.

Besides, don't your needs and desires

change from night to night, week to week, year to year, or minute to minute? That's why it's your responsibility to express your needs on an ongoing basis. Obviously a loving, respectful mate helps. Yet I suspect your level of physical and psychological sophistication is more important, including how well you know your own body, how well you convey your moods and desires, how much you care for your partner, and how secure you feel as a sexual being.

2) The right mind-set is far more influential than knowing the so-called proper techniques. Since good sex is 90 percent mental, how does one go about getting into an intimate state of mind? (I've devoted an entire chapter to this question.) I think the media has done a lot to destroy this whole notion by trying to define *sexy* in a superficial manner. Women especially need to believe that sexy is not based on looks or figure. Men, too. Once a couple internalizes this truth, the sex gets even better.

3) Lastly, a woman needs to be in tune with her physical self. This awareness is crucial. As part of this premise, I include discoveries and explorations with a partner, self-pleasure, and Kegel exercises. Kegels greatly improve a

woman's chance for orgasms by toning up her pubococcygeal (PC) muscle, which works like any other muscle in the body—the more it's used, the stronger it gets. This is covered in more detail in Chapter 5, "Myths About Orgasm."

Friendly Input

During the past seventeen years, I've talked to dozens of women about orgasms. The subject seems to come up every now and then. (Excuse the pun.) Of course, it's also discussed at my seminars, which are designed for this purpose. In any case, I've learned tremendously about sexual proclivities and idiosyncracies through the years.

Over time, as women became more open, sharing many intimate moments, desires, and secrets with me, I reached several striking conclusions:

- Many women do not climax during penetration.
- Most have only one orgasm during sex.
- Some must "work hard" to get that one.
- Many want to climax more easily.

- Most do not own a vibrator.
- Some climax only by oral or manual stimulation.
- Most have not experienced multiple orgasm.
- Many are frustrated by their partner's impatience.
- Some complain about their partner's lack of skill.
- Many women give up too soon in their quest.
- Some opt to fake it rather than make it.

The Good News

I'm not a nymphomaniac or particularly sexy-looking. I'm an average American woman in her thirties who's been fortunate to discover the secret of multiple orgasms. And I want to share my discovery with you. In short, I want you to enjoy the mental, physical, and spiritual dimensions of your sexuality. All in all, it's within reach!

Better still, I believe just about anyone can become orgasmic. You may not be inclined to try everything that's suggested here, and that's okay. We're all different, and I respect your individuality. As you become more knowledgeable through the process of reading or sharing, you're better able to enjoy an enhanced sex life. If you persist in your quest for self-fulfillment, sooner or later you can discover orgasmic paradise!

There's a remarkable benefit to being an orgasmic woman. Not only do you receive a tremendous amount of physical and psychological gratification, but your partner is satisfied by giving you so much pleasure. He starts to think he's the greatest thing since lowfat ice cream. And he is! As his ego swells, he also thinks you're the most fabulous lover in the world! And, with your special man, you are!

The power of love and sexual passion have calmed the forces of man and nature since the beginning of time. The notion of ideal love captivates even the most cynical person once she believes she's found her compatible partner. With its extraordinary power of tenderness and beauty, so the story goes, genuine love tames even the most profane beasts. Personally, I want my man to embody both the beastly lion and the unicorn—symbolic of strength and lust—so I can feel his vitality and his appetite. It's up to all lovers to inspire their mates to treat them compassionately in the bedroom.

The Power of Sex

To be sure, money and prestige are powerful motivators in our society. But never underestimate the power of sex. Sexual love is one of the most profound influences in our lives. Some psychologists claim our second greatest fear is the fear of losing love, coming only behind the fear of losing life itself. Sexual passion can be as powerful as both prestige or money once you learn the secret of *spirited sex*.

Shakespeare once wrote that there's nothing more fragile than the male ego. For some men, there's no greater compliment than to say he's the only one who completely satisfies you in bed. His ability as a lover is reinforced every time you come. So once you become orgasmic, he'll be "under your spell." Trust me, you'll become the unforgettable woman in his life!

The woman who learns how to fully express her passion automatically doubles, or triples, the pleasure of her sex partner. Usually

women are the ones who bring their willingness to express Sentimentality or Tenderness
to a relationship. By contrast, men bring their
willingness to express Strength or Passion. As
you show energy from your heart, your man
opens up to his feelings. Likewise, your partner takes that emotional energy to his primal
core, which awakens your Passion. When a
special bonding takes place, these roles can be
reversed, creating an abundant flow of intense
energy that turns a sexual encounter into
metaphysical bliss!

What Your Mother Never Told You

You may have read about the assorted types
of orgasms, but it really depends on how you
want to classify them. Do you categorize them
based on quality, quantity, or otherwise?
You've probably heard of single, sequential,
and multiple. But have you ever heard of a
perineum or a peritoneal type? How about a
motionless type? Perhaps not. They're lesser
known, more controversial types. Don't worry,
I'd never heard their proper names until later
in life. Often people categorize orgasms as vaginal and clitoral types, which is technically in-

correct. Still others refer to penetration, oral, or manual types.

Recent studies have reported an imagery-based orgasm that doesn't require any physical stimulation. Now, before you scrap the idea, think back. Perhaps you have had one yourself during an erotic dream. In Chapter 5 I discuss various types further for the sake of clarification. In some respects, however, all of these are crude ways of expressing a natural, blissful, and usually intimate experience.

Naturally, I want to tell you up front that I'm not a clinical psychologist, a medical practitioner, or a sex therapist. By choice, I'm a sex educator and an expert at being multiorgasmic. I'll share the marvelous wisdom from ladies who have attended my seminars. Also, I openly reveal what I've experienced on a personal level. Perhaps my book will be different from any other you've read on sexuality because of this unique personal perspective, allowing you a *fly-on-the-wall* view of one woman's sex life.

In brief, this book emphasizes wholesome, *spirited sex*. It focuses on practical, down-to-earth suggestions for better sex and offers helpful insights. While I talk about technique and mechanics to make certain points, that's not my primary educational goal. My genuine mission is to make you think and behave in new or engaging ways. Reconsider how fulfilling your current sex life is, and then act to enhance it in ways that make you feel comfortable.

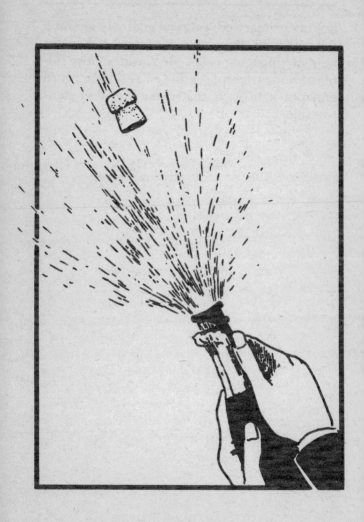

2

Sexually Seize the Day!

Except for winning the lottery, there's no such thing as instant success in anything we try for in life. The professional athlete or dancer spends four to six hours a day training to be considered great. The movie star or comedian who is an "overnight success" may have practiced his or her craft for a dozen years before being *"discovered."* An outstanding teacher is recognized after decades of instruction. Many of us learn how to be competent at a skill or hobby only after years and years of practice.

By contrast, sex therapy tends to get results rather quickly. It also claims to be the most successful type of therapy bar none. Relatively speaking, one can progress a long way in a short time. Reading this book, for example, or talking to a knowledgeable friend about sex can be just as therapeutic, and much less expensive, than a trip to the therapist. Although from time to time, counseling may be necessary.

How many of you saw the movie *Dead Poets Society*? Then you'll recall Robin Williams portrayed an English professor who quoted many great writers. If you had to use two words to describe the theme of that movie, what would they be? Right. *Carpe diem*, which is Horace's Latin for "seize the day." I find it fascinating that most of us try to seize the day when it comes to other challenges in life, like a career, parenting, sports, a religious activity, or a hobby. So why not seize the day when it comes to sex?

Natural as a Sneeze

If sex is a normal part of your life, why not make the most of it? Some folks say I talk about orgasms the way others talk about sneezes. To me, sex is as natural as a sneeze. And, actually, they have a lot in common if you think about it:

a) They're both automatic reflexes.
b) They're both unpredictable.
c) They're both instinctive.
d) They both leave you feeling better.

I just love a good sneeze, don't you? By the way, have you ever stifled a sneeze before? Sure. You've probably controlled one, or attempted to, in a restrictive environment. The same thing can happen with an orgasm if you feel apprehensive or suppressed. Or the opposite can happen: You can open your mind and free yourself for orgasms.

A Frustrated Woman Becomes Orgasmic in Weeks

Now meet Laura MacKenzie, who did just that. An energetic career woman, she fell in love for the first time at the age of twenty-eight. Laura wanted a vaginal (penetration) orgasm more than anything else in the world.

Her lover, Rob, was several years younger and not quite as experienced as Laura in the sexual arena. He had had only two previous lovers. Not that Laura was promiscuous, but in twelve years of dating, she had sexual experiences with a variety of men, though her longest dating stint was only eight months. She'd been able to have orgasms through manual manipulation or oral stimulation. Never did Laura have an orgasm during intercourse.

Hopeful Advice

One fateful evening, Laura and I talked for several hours over a pot of coffee and a pan of homemade brownies. Only once did Laura get close to having a penetration orgasm.

"I almost had one," she told me. "I could tell that something different was happening to me."

"Whaddaya mean?"

"At first, I felt very aroused. It felt great."

"So what happened?" I asked curiously.

"The feeling suddenly went away ... It just vanished, poof."

"Hmmmmmm."

Laura continued, "I felt so frustrated and

letdown that I cried. The poor man looked at me like he'd committed a terrible sin. What's wrong with me?" she asked.

"Nothing is wrong with you," I assured her. "If you were that close, you'll have an orgasm with Rob. I'm sure of it!" My inner voice was talking to me.

I really felt as if I had the answers she needed to get over the orgasmic obstacle. Later we discovered that we liked some of the same things during sex. Eventually Laura and I got into specifics. We trusted each other enough to keep these details confidential. One thing lead to another, and soon I had told her a number of things I did that had worked for me.

Two and a half weeks after our chat, Laura came over with a bottle of brut champagne in hand. "I did it!" she exclaimed gleefully.

"Did what?" I asked excitedly.

"I had a penetration orgasm with Rob!"

"I'm so happy for you!" I said.

Her face was flush and her eyes twinkled as she talked. "You really helped get me over the hump." We both laughed.

"Sometimes it just takes a little information," I added.

"I'll never to be able to thank you enough,"

she said, "but here's a token of my appreciation." She handed me the champagne.

I glowed with pride as I accepted her earnest gift. "Perhaps I've found my niche in life," I said jokingly. "I think I'll become a sex adviser." Perhaps the bud of an idea was born that day, which eventually blossomed into this manual. I'd like to think so.

Informal Survey Results

I surveyed one hundred women in the San Francisco Bay Area to see if their experiences were anything like Laura's. All respondents were between the ages of twenty and fifty-five, and from a variety of economic and ethnic backgrounds. For this handful of questions, the results were revealing:

Question—Do you have orgasms through intercourse on a regular basis?
38 said "Yes."
53 said "No."
9 said "Sometimes."

Question—Do you engage in oral sex, either as the recipient or the giver?

85 said "Yes."
12 said "No."
3 didn't answer the question.

Question—Have you ever had a multiple or sequential orgasm through intercourse?
15 said "Yes."
67 said "No."
18 were confused or declined to answer.

Question—Would you like to learn how to have multiple orgasms?
49 said "Yes."
33 said "No."
18 said "Not applicable."
(A few said it would scare them)

Question—If there were one thing you could change about your current partner's skill in bed, what would that be?
26 said "Nothing."
58 said "More foreplay."
16 gave varied answers:
   to verbalize needs more
   to agree on the time of day
   to decrease the frequency
   to increase the frequency
   to hug more afterward

Humans are very enigmatic, like a riddle. While some women were extremely candid in their answers and wanted to discuss more issues, others were obviously uncomfortable with the subject matter. Even though the questionnaire was confidential (names were not even requested), some didn't want to share personal information. Some women refused to fill out the complete form. A few wrote in funny answers to almost every question. Too much joking suggests that they were uncomfortable with the material and may have used humor as a defense mechanism.

There is no right or wrong here, but I think sexually active adults need to come to grips with their sexuality. In light of the current AIDS crisis, we must be able to discuss it openly and maturely with our partners and our children. Most important, we must be honest with ourselves in order to experience lifelong pleasure.

Where Do You Fit Into the Puzzle?

3

Sexiness Is Mental

Sexiness has nothing to do with your looks or your figure. It has everything to do with your mind! Trust me, being sexy is 90 percent mental and 10 percent physical. Haven't you ever gone out with a man who looks like a Greek god, adorned with a perfectly square jaw, tan and gorgeous, only to find out that he kisses like a brick? Then he proceeds to talk about himself until you're nauseated, and he never asks for your impression of anything. To top it off, you mention you like Mozart, and he asks if they're a new group. The old cliché *you can't judge a book by its cover* is true in this regard.

Time and time again I hear women exclaim, "Hey, get a load of the hunk I've been going out with lately" when they show someone a photo of their current lover. Sure it's natural to comment on a nice pair of buns every now and then, but our society is obsessed by physical appearances to the exclusion of other, more important, traits. If you can't look at another man without wondering how he looks nude or how good he is in bed, seek professional help.

We complain that men treat us like pieces of meat, and then some of us do the same thing in reverse. As Joan Rivers would say, "Oh, grow up!" Feel free to admire what was given to the male of the species by a power greater than humans, then get to know the person inside the body before assuming he's the best catch of the decade. As you know, many men who are strikingly handsome seem to think they're "God's gift to women" and consequently become shallow, self-serving, manipulative womanizers or worse. Naturally, there are exceptions to the rule.

To be truly sexy, a person has to have a genuine affection and respect for the opposite sex. You've met the type. He's the man who has that indescribable twinkle in his eye, the man who makes you feel special, the man who freely gives a sense of love, possibly a feeling you've never experienced before. Remember, by being loved, you become more lovable. And the more you make him feel special, the more sensual he becomes. So the cycle continues. It's a two-way street to paradise. As a result, both people become better lovers, and, hopefully, better friends.

Is Your Man the Sir Lancelot or the King Arthur Type?

I have a theory about decent men—those who treat women well—that I want to share. I believe there are basically two types of good men: 1) the *Sir Lancelot* type and 2) the *King Arthur* type. Most of us grew up dreaming about Sir Lancelot, who comes and sweeps us off our feet by whispering sweet nothings in our ears. Although we typically visualize an extremely handsome man, it doesn't really matter what he looks like, because this type never lacks for words. He will write you poetry and compare you to the four seasons or make elaborate analogies about his love for you. He will not only send you flowers, but pick them himself.

He's complimentary (even if it stretches our

imagination); he's attentive and faithful (even when you ask for some personal space); he's very loving and supportive. These Sir Lancelot types put women on a pedestal (whether or not we deserve it); they almost treat us like we're not human. Now, it's easy to fall in love with a man who's totally devoted to you. And so you love this man even if you're not compatible on other levels—intellectual, spiritual, social, emotional, academic, career, and family. If you are actually in harmony with a man like this, treat him with the same respect he shows you. Above all, love him well in return.

Now, the King Arthur types, by comparison, may seem a little dull. But let's not judge them too harshly. These men will probably never write you poetry or pick flowers for you, but they can be very steady, self-reliant mates. While they may appear a bit detached when you're out in public, they save all their passion for the bedroom. A trade-off worth more than diamonds and rubies, in my opinion.

King Arthur types are also devoted to their women, but it's demonstrated in a more subtle, less flamboyant manner than Sir Lancelot. He will stand by his mate in all sorts of personal weather. Since he sees things in black and white, he is unable to exaggerate the truth to spare your feelings. If you ask him what he thinks about the new outfit you bought, beware. He'll tell you the truth. (The more tactful types will say, "Whatever you think is best, dear.") But the message is clear just the same. At least you can always count on his honesty. So if he says, "I love you," you can bet that he means it. Naturally, that's more valuable than a thousand pseudo-Lancelots.

If you haven't found your true Sir Lancelot, maybe it's because you've already got a King Arthur type. Appreciate what you have and stop looking elsewhere!

The Confusion Between Sexy and Sensual

We're bombarded by media-made images that tell us how we're supposed to look, talk, smell, feel, act, and even love. Consequently we have a superficial sense of what it means to be sexy. After all, commercials are trying to sell us a product. Of course, they'll brainwash you to think you have to have it to attract the opposite sex. While some products are necessary, many cover up our natural attractiveness. Don't you think that a healthy, inherent smell is twice as appealing as half the products on the market today?

We need to keep life in the proper perspective by not being so vulnerable to the media's idea of the perfect mate...which reminds me of a quick story. Before my twin sister got married a few years ago, she used to date quite a bit. Every month or so she'd tell me, "Yeah, I was out last night trying to find the perfect man."

I'd always respond on cue, "Did you find him?"

"Sure, I found him," she said. "The only trouble was, he was looking for the perfect woman." The pathetic irony, of course, is that many women search for the perfect mate. He doesn't really exist. And neither does the perfect woman. If more women learned to embrace their mates for who and what they are, we'd be a lot happier in our relationships.

To help keep a balance, then, let's turn to the dictionary. Webster defines SEXY as "sexually suggestive and stimulating; erotic." It defines SENSUAL as "relating to the gratification of the senses or an indulgence of appetite."

As you see, each word has a slightly different meaning. You've undoubtedly known a "touchy" person—perhaps you are one yourself—someone who enjoys holding hands or hugging easily. You tend to be labeled as flirtatious or sensual, right? Or do you indulge other appetites like eating, drinking, dancing, and sunbathing? If you are a touchy person, you're probably more willing to try new things with a sex partner because of your natural desire for pleasing the senses. You may be close to a more satisfying sexual experience. If you're not a touchy person, this book can still guide you toward an enhanced sex life if you give it half a chance.

So What Characterizes Sexiness?

Don't you agree that *sexiness* is a state of mind? Wouldn't you want the man in your life to have certain qualities? Of course, this works both ways. Women, too, should strive for a blend of these same qualities. I believe being sexy encompasses six basic characteristics:

1) Self-confidence/Balance
2) Affectionate/Tender
3) Successful/Productive
4) Humorous/Witty/Fun
5) Energetic/Healthy
6) Attentive/Responsive

1) A man with a healthy ego and a good sense of self-esteem is invariably sexy. As you know, someone who talks constantly about himself usually has the opposite problem: low self-esteem. He's a bore in the long run. Who wants to live with that on a daily basis?

Ask a man to describe himself in ten or more adjectives and then count how many are negative. If more than 30 percent are negative, he probably doesn't have a very high self-esteem. And overconfidence is likewise distasteful—if he answers with 100 percent perfect traits. There's a thin line between being self-assured and being cocky. Balance is the key word here.

Give me a Renaissance man any day.

If a man carries himself well, is conversational in a variety of subjects (not just sports and business), is fairly intelligent, considerate, and attentive, don't you find him irresistible? A truly self-assured man comes across in the bedroom as gentle, caring, and thoughtful. He has no need to demonstrate a macho attitude; he doesn't think of women as a mere conquest. He likes himself; and he's relaxed around the opposite sex.

Remember, it takes a really strong person to admit he or she is unsure once in a while.

Perhaps your relationship is on the brink of being redefined. Are you discussing the possibility of living together, being monogamous, making a commitment, or dating other people? That may be a confusing time for both parties. So if a man tells you he feels a little insecure about your relationship, accept his feelings as real, and listen to what he has to say. Don't shut him off with quick-fix statements like "Oh, you know I love you." Ask him why he feels that way. Then listen some more.

If a man thinks you'll stay with him no matter how badly he treats you, dump him! He's either too cocky for his own good or he's got a personality disorder. Perhaps he's an underground woman hater (someone who puts you on a pedestal in public, but privately humiliates you) or he's got a terrible inferiority complex, or both.

2) An affectionate man is worth his weight in gold. As you know, there's a big difference between the guy who's touchy in public, yet only wants his needs met in bed, and the truly affectionate man. If you're honest with yourself, you know the difference instinctively. Personally, I'd rather have a gentleman in public and a stud in bed any day! Wouldn't you rather have a man who likes to be around you as a

person? Then his sexual touch becomes penetratingly passionate and stimulating. There's a warmer quality to a loving touch than one that's merely mechanically correct.

Equally important to being touched sensually is a person who has the same level of desire for you as you do for him. You can't put a price on a characteristic like that! This trait can last a lifetime with the right person and only a few weeks with the wrong one. Don't you agree it's more special than most people think? If one person is always the initiator, it can take away from the experience for the other person. While men are brought up to be the sexual aggressor, more and more women today are expressing their desires and getting good results. A secure man enjoys being the seducee periodically. Each couple has to work out what's right and comfortable.

Matching sexual appetites will be discussed further in Chapter 8. Passion begins with true fondness. Don't you want a man who has a genuine warm desire for you? It doesn't have to be an animalistic, overwhelming passion that never seems to go away. And it doesn't have to be a man who wants you every day either. In fact, that may be a sign of a sex addict. Don't you love it when your mate gives you a fond, sweet pat on your buns as he passes by you in the hallway? Don't you savor it best when it's least expected ... like when you've just finished mopping the kitchen floor or changed the oil in your car? True affection is the glue that holds together a solid relationship. As the affection goes, so goes the relationship.

3) Most women agree success is sexy. Some mistakenly believe success is related to the size of a man's wallet, however, without giving consideration to other characteristics. But, remember, what constitutes success for one person may not for another! Success is subjective. Most people connect it with material possessions or the amount of money someone has accumulated, but actually it's the accomplishment of whatever goal someone decides is worthwhile. As long as the man is productive, is able to support himself and his children, he's acceptable.

Just as each woman has her own journey to fulfill, so does a man. For most people, a well-balanced life is desired; others must become an expert in a specialized field before they consider themselves triumphant. To be reasonably happy and fulfilled in one's work, one's hobbies, and one's personal life is to be successful. Enough said.

4) A marvelous sense of humor goes a long

way. The couple who laughs, lasts. This may be more important than sex itself. (And it takes a lot for me to say that!) Honestly, don't you agree that someone who makes you laugh outside of bed is more likely to please you in bed? Sex should be playful. If we take ourselves too seriously, we lose the spontaneity of the moment. It's also harder to relax if we take the act of sex too somberly or analyze it to death. I like to have fun in bed.

I recall one episode with my partner when our regular smooth routine turned into a comedy of errors. For whatever reason, we just weren't in sync. I'd turn one way just as he'd pivot another, or we'd move our arms at the same time only to get tangled up. When I was ready for penetration, he wasn't. Well, you get the picture. Before either of us became too frustrated, I decided to say something. Just as I opened my mouth, my partner said, "Let's try our luck at origami; I think we'd have a better chance at that tonight." That broke the tension and we ended up chuckling about it. We decided to take a break. After snuggling and talking for an half hour, we worked up the passion again. This time, everything was fantastic as usual.

In short, a warm smile and genuine laughter go a long way with most women. Woody Allen once said "sex is the most fun anyone can have without laughing." With or without laughter, it's the most fun I've ever had!

5) Most women concur that a healthy man is sexy. Now, the picture of health doesn't necessarily mean a well-tanned six-foot-two-inch, 195-pound athletic type. Health equals energy, and energy is a turn-on. Most women want a man who takes care of himself—someone who eats healthful food, drinks in moderation if at all, exercises, and sleeps well on a regular basis. He doesn't have to be a marathon runner, just take reasonably good care of himself. I respect that, don't you?

Besides, I play racquetball and work out at the club several times a week myself. I deserve someone who likes aching muscles as much as I do. If you're physically active, perhaps you desire a fitness nut (I mean athlete). You two deserve each other. The couple who works out together, lasts. There's probably more truth to that statement than meets the eye. I've seen many sturdy, energetic seasoned citizens holding hands and walking together or, more recently, snow-skiing together. I always get a warm spot in my heart for people who obviously enjoy their partner's companionship in sports.

6) Last, but not least, an attentive man is

sexy. We all need to feel appreciated. No matter how smart or pretty or successful you are, you still need to be reinforced (for those thousand other deeds you do on your journey to becoming the finest person you can be). Verbal praise goes a long way toward making a relationship last.

When your partner is responsive to your needs, both spoken and unspoken, don't you feel loved? While we shouldn't expect our mates to read our minds, we can require them to respect our wishes. For instance, if we ask our partner not to tell a particular story or joke at a friend's house, he should honor our request. A responsive man is generally in touch with his own feelings, which allows him to be sympathetic to another person's emotions.

Generally speaking, he perceives himself to be part of a Universal Connectedness. This may sound a little out in left field for some of you. But I like a man who realizes there is more to life than just what the senses are able to perceive. If he lacks a spiritual dimension, he lacks depth, insight, and the ability to understand life's cycle of birth, death, rebirth.

The so-called trivial activities of life count as well. When a man really listens to our opinions, new ideas we've encountered, our constantly changing impressions of life or basic chatter of the day, it shows us he cares. We, in turn, owe our partners the same attention and positive response. A platonic friend of mine recently told me that I knew more about him than his second wife, a woman he lived with for nearly ten years. "How can that be?" I asked curiously. "I've only known you for six months."

"You ask questions about my day and then you listen to me."

"Of course I do, but that's simple."

"It obviously wasn't for her."

The point is, if you care about someone, listen to him on a regular basis. Most of us don't demand to be *understood,* just *heard.* My hunch is that many extramarital affairs sprout out of the need to be listened to. Stop and think about it, and then LISTEN, LISTEN, LISTEN.

There's an old joke about a woman who began complaining to her hairdresser about her husband of twenty-three years and threatened to leave the ole *stick-in-the-mud.*

The cosmetologist made one simple request. "Do me a favor, Vera; compliment your husband at least twice a day for the next month."

"Are you crazy?" the wife replied. "Haven't you been listening to a word I've said?"

"Do it for me."

"All right," she agreed reluctantly.

At Vera's next hair appointment, her hairdresser asked if she'd left her husband yet.

"Are you crazy?" came the reply. "He's the sweetest man in the world!" Pay attention to your man, and he will most likely be responsive to your needs. Again, it's a two-way street to paradise.

To sum up, someone who is self-assured, funny, energetic, attentive, and successful is likely to turn women on. If your partner has those attributes and shows true passion on a regular basis, then it's a match made in heaven! What attracts us to another human being is sometimes a mystery, but many women agree with these basics. Think about it. What do you consider sexy?

Now that you have all the sexy answers, go out and seize the day!

4

The Right Mind-set

Okay, you're on your way to internalizing the belief that sexiness is 90 percent mental and you embrace *sex-equity lovemaking*. Still, how do you actually become an equal, compatible sex partner? A loving and respectful mate helps, but more important is your progression to the realization you're becoming the finest individual you can be. A journey worth taking at any age. Even with your special mate, some days it's hard to find the energy and wind down from the day. Essentially, how do you get into the right frame of mind for sex when career, finances, kids, community obligations, or the daily hubbub of life get in the way? Well, that's what this chapter is all about.

First, find out how sensuous you are. Choose the most appropriate response to the following ten questions. By taking this short quiz, you'll see where you fit in. Then use the information as a springboard to discovering your personal journey to heightened sexual pleasure.

Sensuality Self-Quiz

1) **When you first went out with your partner, you:**

   a) Kept your distance because you'd been hurt before

   b) Liked his physical features right away and couldn't keep your hands off him

   c) Couldn't wait to talk to him to find out more about him

   d) Waited to see if he was attracted to you before pursuing a deeper relationship

2) **If time wasn't a factor, how would you wash yourself?**

   a) Prefer a quick shower using a washcloth

   b) Prefer a shower putting soap on directly

   c) Take a regular bath and use a washcloth

   d) Take a long, hot bath and put soap directly on your skin

3) When you kiss someone you care for, you usually:

a) Think about your grocery list or something else you have to do in the near future

b) Wish he'd move on, so you can get to the real stuff

c) Try to impress him with your technique

d) Enjoy the sensations for themselves

4) When thinking back to what attracted you to your lover, you:

a) Think about his physique

b) Think about his hair

c) Think about his facial features

d) Think about his scent

5) How would you describe your activity level?

a) It's unladylike to sweat, so I'd rather watch than participate in sports

b) I prefer activities such as gardening, reading, handcrafts

c) I like a mixture of sports—walking, horseback riding, etc.

d) I participate in aerobic sports like

swimming or racquetball on a regular basis

6) **While making love, how would you best describe your style?**

   a) I usually let him take the lead, and I follow

   b) I assert myself verbally to tell him how to meet my needs

   c) I take the lead intermittently, and he follows

   d) I prefer a natural mixture of who leads and who follows

7) **Which of the following applies most to you while making love?**

   a) I'm rather reserved and quiet

   b) I prefer being on the bottom—it's less work

   c) I prefer to be on top or sideways—work is fun

   d) A mixture of fast/slow, tough/tender, etc., is best

8) **When dining at a fine restaurant, you usually:**

   a) Order the same thing over and over—food is food

b) I'd rather be safe than sorry, so I ask for the waiter's recommendation

c) I focus mainly on who I'm with and enjoy the atmosphere

d) I try to savor the taste of new and exotic foods

9) **You're at the beach or park on a sunny spring day; you:**

a) Feel uncomfortable and hot

b) Would rather be inside or in the shade

c) Enjoy the fresh air for itself

d) Feel right at home

10) **You're at a party, and everyone there has a common interest. You've just met an attractive man who is new to the group; you:**

a) Freeze up and wait for him to talk to you

b) Want to impress him, but you just can't think of anything clever to say at the moment

c) Talk to him as you would anyone else you've seen at the party (after introducing yourself)

d) Discuss your mutual interest, curious for his response

To score yourself, simply count up the number of A's, B's, C's, and D's that you have, and write that in the space below:

A _____ B _____ C _____ D _____

What Your Score Means

If mostly A's: Becoming sensual is not on the top of your priority list. You'd rather work than pamper yourself. You're more interested in other things in your life right now. Still, you can refocus your energies into this area if desired. Once you indulge yourself, you'll realize the benefits. Why not use this quiz as a starting point? By all means, read the rest of this manual and begin treating yourself, as well as the special man in your life.

If mostly B's: Your prognosis for becoming sensual is fair. Though without the suit of armor of the person above, you seem to have analytical ideas on what sensuality is all about. You may only need to find the confidence to move on to greater sources of pleasure for yourself and your mate. If you manage to break out of your feet-on-the-ground mold, you'll find many rewards. Soaking in a tub is not a waste of time. It's relaxing. Perhaps you just need more time to explore your own sensuality and expand your horizons.

If mostly C's: This score indicates a good chance for physical and emotional fulfillment. You're obviously comfortable with the senses and their rewards. The touch of fur, silk, or warm water on your body is exciting. You enjoy feeling desirable to the opposite sex. You appreciate pleasurable experiences. You're to be commended. I have a hunch that sensual paradise is at your doorstep!

If mostly D's: Bravo! No doubt you're the perfect picture of sensuality to your mate (or yourself). Things could hardly be better. You're willing to try new things in your romance and in your life. Keep up the good work! The outlook for a lifetime of fulfilling sex is great. If not already there, it's on the horizon. Men find you tantalizing! They want to join you in your zest for life!

Self-Esteem in the Bedroom

Does Self-Esteem Play a Role in How You React with Your Partner?

You bet! Nobody can separate self-esteem from his or her personal experiences in or out of bed. It only makes sense that the more confident you are about who you are, the better lover you'll make. When you're sure of yourself, aren't you more willing to try new things? Wouldn't you be more likely to make advances when you're in the mood? An insecure person would be afraid of rejection. The secure person could handle an honest reply such as "I appreciate the invitation, but I'm too tired right now."

Remember it's also important to be tactful if you're the one saying no. "Could I rest up first? It's been a long day," for example, is not an out-and-out rejection, but rather a delay of the inevitable. Some couples have created personalized phrases to make the point:

- My heart's in the right place, but the body ain't able.

- Can I take a rain check, please?

- Could we cuddle instead tonight?

- I'm in the neighborhood, but I'm not there yet.

- You'll be the first to know, honey, I promise.

- You were so overwhelming the last time, I don't feel the need just yet.

You get the idea. Your partner shouldn't make you feel guilty when you say no, and vice versa. That's a sign of an ill-fated relationship.

On the other hand, if your mate rarely or never initiates, there's a problem as well. Both extremes are unhealthy.

Does Your Partner Make You Feel Special in and Out of Bed?

A man once said, "All women are lovely when they make love!" This Sir Lancelot type truly loves women and makes us feel beautiful. And when it's genuine, there's no comparable feeling. Never underestimate the power of a woman's intuition. I believe that most females instinctively know when a man is feeding them a line and when it's sincere.

Have you ever felt that warm glow when your partner spontaneously gives you a squeeze while you're watching TV? When his touch becomes an unconscious gesture, it becomes even more special. A visual man may prefer going places, doing activities together, or buying things to show how much he loves a woman. Auditory men would rather talk to their sweethearts or say it with music. Given a choice, kinesthetic males favor staying home and making love. Now, I prefer an all-around gentleman who likes a combination of these traits. (In Chapter 8 I'll discuss how to enhance communication—sexually and otherwise—with each type of man.)

To feel special is to feel a toasty blush inside. I get my best warm fuzzies in the bedroom. Whatever has transpired during the rest of the day, let the world go by once you engage in sex. From his initial kiss, put yourself into the *right psychological mind-set* by being totally absorbed in the moment. This can actually be practiced, I believe, alone or with your partner. According to Anthony Robbins in his book *Unlimited Power,* you can actually put yourself into a loving state of mind . . . depending on which operational mode is your predominant style—visual, auditory, or kinesthetic. First, ask yourself this question:

What one thing is absolutely necessary for me to feel totally loved?

Do you have to *see* a certain look in your lover's face? Do you have to *hear* particular words in a distinct tone of voice? Or do you have to be *touched* a specific way? Once you discover the real answer to this, your lover can put you into "state" virtually any time by recreating the response you require to feel totally loved. This simple trigger sets off a complex series of messages to your central nervous system. Human beings are basically programmed by past intense experiences. And, if you're smart, you can reuse these "anchors" to trigger positive and loving responses over and over again.

By the way, have you said or done anything lately to show your mate that he's unique? When was the last time you wrote a provocative note or sent a card or complimented your mate for his lovable nature? When was the last time you sent him flowers for that remarkably sensual romp by the fireplace?

Does Your Mate Compare You To Past Lovers?

I hope not. I may be old-fashioned, but I don't want to hear a single thing about past lovers other than a general comment such as "They don't hold a candle to you." Details only create problems. Even if something is said in passing, casually, it can be taken out of context and exaggerated in the mind of the other person. Let's say your current partner tells you he was once with this amazing woman who never, ever got tired of sex ... She could go on for hours ... It was unbelievable. If you currently average thirty minutes, you might end up feeling second-rate. In the back of your mind, there'd be a haunting image of a nameless woman who gave your mate more pleasure than he could endure.

Now, the truth of the matter could be that he didn't enjoy the lovemaking because he felt too pressured to perform for long periods of time, and he feels much more comfortable and relaxed with you. But perhaps the conversation got cut off before the whole truth was discussed. Some things are better left unsaid— even between spouses—and details of past sexual affairs is one of them, in my opinion.

Of course, this works both ways. For instance, if you told your mate that your ex-husband used to drive you crazy (in a positive sense) by licking your neck, don't you think that puts undue pressure on your lover? Except for a rare man, your partner would be less likely to continue that tradition for fear of ending up on the short end by comparison. It's a sticky wicket. Make it a rule in your relationship to never speak of past details. Steer clear of undesirable hurdles. The best way to express your desires is to use a phrase that doesn't make a comparison in the first place, such as, "You'd make me crazy if you'd lick my neck a little."

How Do You Perceive YOUR Own Body?

Unfortunately, many women have a negative attitude about their bodies—even if they're above average in attractiveness. This happens in many ways. The media, for one, typically holds up so-called perfect models (usually too thin) as what we should strive to look like. A friend or family member, intentionally or unintentionally, may have made fun of a certain part of our anatomy during a crucial time in our upbringing. Women carry these negative ideas in their heads long after they're not true anymore. During my adolescence, my boyfriend called me "bird legs." It took me years to appreciate the attractiveness of my slender legs.

We need to come to the point where we can honestly say to ourselves:

"I'm comfortable inside my body...It's the only one I've ever known...I've worn this frame a long time...It may not be perfect, but it works for me."

Respect for the body needs to flow both ways. Don't make your partner feel bad over being too short, too tall, too large, too thin. Nothing's wrong with encouragement to be healthy, but nagging or name calling goes too far. How we talk about our bodies can enhance or detract from a sexual experience. Be careful. Words flung today could be tomorrow's regret.

Have You Ever Been in a Long-Distance Relationship?

Most of us have been separated from the man we love for an extended period of time— say two or more months. Don't you remember the great sex you had when you finally met on those special weekends? Didn't anticipation play a part in your enjoyment? Shouldn't it still play a role? If so, how can you recreate a sense of anticipatory excitement now that you're married or live together or live in the same city? After these self-assessing questions, I offer two dozen practical suggestions for doing just that.

- Do you periodically take the time to dress up and look as presentable now as you did during your long-distance affair?

- Did you think about sex for two to three days prior to your visits so that you had practically worked up a lather by the time you saw each other?

- Did you talk on the telephone, sometimes for hours, about what you planned to do when you saw each other?

- Did you buy little gifts to exchange with each other back then, and dropped the habit now that you live together or live in the same town?

- What other differences are there that may unconsciously perpetuate your taking each other a bit for granted now compared to then?

Twenty-four Practical Solutions for Getting the Right Mind-set

Naturally, this list is not meant as a panacea to correct deeper problems in a relationship. It's meant as suggestions for couples who want to synchronize their passion for lovemaking. Because of hectic schedules and life-styles, it's more difficult for couples to be in a sexual mood at the same time these days. Perhaps this will kindle a few seductive ideas of your own.

Ideas to Do by Yourself:

1) Read an erotic passage from your favorite book (or trashy novel).
2) Place a dozen candles all around the bathroom while you take a long, sultry bath with sweet-smelling oils or bubbles.

Shave your legs with luxurious soap, and use buffing cream or a sponge all over your body for a smooth finish.

3) Give yourself a facial. Use a commercial mask if available. Otherwise, egg whites will do the trick. Try avocado if you desire. And why stop with just your face? If you feel like it, put it all over your body.

4) Get yourself a pedicure, if affordable, or do your own toenails. Then massage your feet, especially your ankle area (an erotic zone).

5) Have a cup of hot tea or glass of wine and listen to soul-basic music by Aretha Franklin or whatever else flips your switch.

6) Write a provocative message on your mate's mirror in lipstick or put a note on his pillow: *"I love ya like the devil! That's why I'm gonna screw the hell outta ya!"*

7) Go to a museum with famous photographs, paintings, sculptures; then let your mind wander. You'll be amazed at your creative digressions.

8) Dress in sexy lingerie under your work clothes. Your subconscious mind will automatically muse about sex throughout your workday.

9) Rent an erotic movie and watch your favorite scene over and over.

10) Go directly to the monkey/gorilla enclosures at your local zoo.

11) Lay quietly on satin sheets for thirty minutes (I call this *libido meditation*).

12) Use your vibrator (or hand) and fantasize about your partner.

Ideas to Do with Your Partner:

1) Sunbathe together, briefly, then draw a bath for your mate and tell him something sweet about what attracted you to him when you first met.

2) Put on that special tune—the one playing when you fell in love—and ask your partner to dance with you. Make it a fun thing to do, not a duty.

3) Do a relaxation technique together, such as deep breathing, and try to match your pace for three to five min-

utes. If you know any Yoga, try an exercise or two.

4) If atmosphere elevates your mood, then have a candlelight dinner, a glass of wine by the fireplace, music, or turn down the lights and just sit together.

5) To unwind, try playing a game in bed—your favorite card game, Yatzee, Trivial Pursuit, or Boggle. The mood may strike sooner than you think.

6) Meet your partner at a single's place and make believe you've just met. Start out at opposite ends of the bar, for example, and eventually make your way over. Pretend you're from another city and have a different career.

7) Recreate the first conversation you two had together by going back to where you first met, if possible. If not, go to a similar place.

8) Change venues. If you can afford it, take a minivacation every other month to get reacquainted outside your normal surroundings. Even if money is tight, you can always go to a park (after hours) and have a private picnic. Select

a romantic place. Or switch houses with some friends in a similar situation.

9) Burn some incense and use some aromatic oils for a foot or back massage to set the mood. Each person deserves at least ten uninterrupted minutes.

10) Put a dozen or so candles around your bedroom and bask in the ambience.

11) You could spice up the routine by role-playing. Pretend to be someone else. (Make up a character.) Become Christine, for instance, the sophisticated lady who is very aggressive sexually. Then go the opposite route and play a terribly shy woman, Sabrina, who needs to be shown the romantic ropes.

12) Determine what gets you into "a loving state of mind." Figure out if you need visual, auditory, or kinesthetic stimulation from your mate, in what dosages, and how often to keep feeling loved. Most important, anchor these positive feelings in the bedroom. (More on this in Chapter 8.)

Good luck! Hopefully, some of these ideas will set some sparks flying.

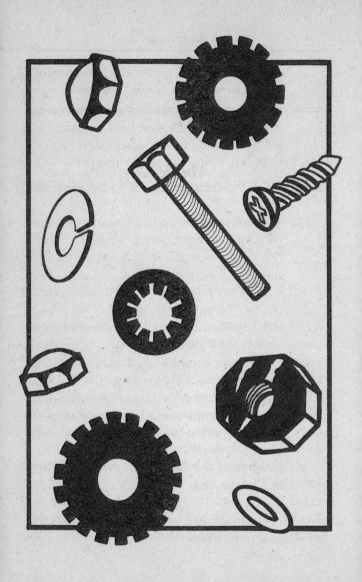

5

Myths About Orgasm

There exists a whole host of myths and misconceptions that we buy into even if we aren't
conscious we believe them. These unexamined
assumptions may dictate our practices. And
even if we make resolutions that we're going
to change, we usually don't. Behavior experts
claim it takes between twenty-one and forty
days to create a new habit; and apparently this
only occurs when we make a concerted effort
to make a specific change.

When we have a belief, it affects our behavior patterns. In fact, one belief is more powerful than one thousand good intentions.
Realistically, our past experiences associated
with sex are a combination of both positive and

negative episodes. If your experiences are negative because of a thoughtless or crude partner, then you may decide all men are self-oriented. If you've been physically violated, the belief may be more deeply ingrained.

Since we live in a stimulus-response world, our sexual behavior is very dependent on past encounters. Some women require counseling to untangle the web of dreadful negativity imprinted on their minds; others need to rethink their original beliefs; and a lucky few are simply looking to discover deeper and richer ways to express their love.

What are some of the myths and misconceptions that dominate us?

1) That clitoral and vaginal orgasms are two separate types
2) That some orgasms are artificial or wicked
3) That various types of orgasms are fraudulent
4) That the stages of arousal prior to orgasm are contrived
5) That Kegel exercises are only for sex fiends

There are other myths, of course, but I choose to examine these five issues. The next two chapters will discuss additional myths. There's enough misinformation about the particulars associated with climaxing that I wanted to devote this entire chapter to it. I hope this clarifies some of the mystery.

What Exactly Is an Orgasm?

Before we go into the first myth, let's define orgasm as: *an automatic reflex that happens once the body, particularly the clitoris, has been adequately stimulated, and is expressed by vaginal contractions.* No matter what prompts it, it's the same physiologically. Just as a rose cannot be called by any other name, an orgasm is an orgasm is an orgasm. Still, roses come in a variety of colors, shapes, and sizes.

The Clitoral/Vaginal Misconception

The clitoral-versus-vaginal-orgasm controversy is an imperfect anatomical way of explaining a difference. It's an inane controversy in terms of the physiology of an orgasm. Clinical research has shown that there is no orgasm without tactile friction applied directly or indirectly to the clitoris. So, technically, it is incorrect to say "vaginal" orgasm. If you want to refer to the source of stimulation, I suggest you say *penetration-stimulated* orgasm (or, at least, the abbreviated version, *penetration orgasm,* which I'll use throughout the book).

In spite of the fact that most orgasms are physiologically identical, the feelings associated with them tend to be different. That's because the reflex of an orgasm has both a motor and a sensory component. The motor, or physical, presentation is expressed by contractions in and around the vagina. The sensory, or feeling, expression is the location of the trigger of the reflex.

The Seed of Arousal

Let's face it, women have orgasms by four basic sources of stimulation:

a) By manual manipulation
b) By oral stimulation
c) By vaginal penetration
d) By anal excitation

To say any of these is artificial, contrived, or wicked is a misconception; the second type may be against certain people's religious practices; the fourth type may be unconventional, but some women swear by them. Anal intercourse is not my cup of tea, but who am I to say what two consenting adults should or shouldn't do privately? Enough said.

Facts and Feelings

With the knowledge we now have available, I encourage women to use more accurate terms when discussing orgasms. Why not use *manually stimulated, orally stimulated, penetration-stimulated,* or *anally stimulated orgasm?*

- Manually stimulated orgasms have many variations, including use of finger or hand, use of a vibrator, and use of other objects or parts of the body for stimulation. To be specific, one could say, "I had a Jacuzzi-stimulated orgasm." (Try it, you may like it.)

  With manual stimulation, especially during masturbation, orgasm feels as intense as women desire, because direct contact on the clitoris can make it unbearably pleasurable. But there's little depth to them, no guts, no emotional impact. Mainly physical release. Many women find them to be much more intense than penetration orgasms, but I've discovered that there can be the same level of intensity with other methods.

- Through oral stimulation, orgasms seem smooth, soft, powerful, or intense, depending on your mate's technique. There's a warmth and pressure on the genital area that cannot be matched by any other means of manipulation. Cunnilingus feels marvelously primitive and basic, intimate in a special way. Granted it's fairly common for women to have multiple or sequential orgasms in cunnilingus, but this book focuses on the next category.

- With a penetration orgasm, many women feel a more diffused, softer, gentler sensation. I would have agreed with that until my late twenties when I discovered I could have just as spasmodic and intense an orgasm through intercourse as during masturbation or oral sex. Sometimes, after a particularly arousing round of foreplay, I'm able to experience an orgasm within seconds after penetration. Usually I feel a slow building up of tension that starts in a core spot inside my vagina, and extends outward like the ripples in a pond after tossing a stone into the water. Suddenly it's like the entire dam breaks and the pressure is relieved. Technically speaking, that's what happens as the blood surrounding the vaginal wall is built up and then released during climax.

- Anally stimulated orgasm seems to be of two types: external and internal, where the clitoris is somehow getting indirect pressure. An internally stimulated one has been described to me as all-consuming, erupting from a potent core within the body and extending outward. A few women say there's no sensation quite like it, and in fact, they crave the explosive nature of it. Others claim to be neutral, while several assert it was simply a onetime experimental interlude that they don't care to repeat. An externally stimulated type can be very explosive as well, and can happen more than once.

Let's talk about how an orgasm feels. See if this has a ring of familiarity. Many women have described an orgasm as:

- rejuvenating, energizing, electrifying
- palpitating, engulfing, overflowing
- moist hotness, titillating
- erupting pleasure, fulfilling
- pulsating feeling in the vagina
- a profound twitching sensation
- being on the brink of an earthquake

However you describe it, it's a positively wonderful feeling. Agreed? (If you've never experienced one, read on. It'll happen sooner than you think.) For me, an orgasmic experience is deep, oceanic, magical...and metaphysical when I can't tell where my body stops and his starts. Frequently it reaches a spiritual level. Why else do women say, "oh, God...oh, oh" during climax? Joking aside, I believe that sex connects us to an otherworldly feeling. As ancient Judaic writings of the Talmud say, "Sex is a foretaste of the world to come."

Ways to Classify Orgasms

As I alluded to in Chapter 1, cataloging orgasms is subjective because it depends on how you approach the process. You can base it on the source of stimulation, which has been discussed in generic terms, or base it on quality, which is an individual preference, or base it on the quantity and timing concept, which is one of the simplest ways to classify orgasms:

1) Single
2) Multiple
3) Sequential

Additional types could be considered a variation, or subcategory, of any of those: the internally *peritoneal-stimulated* or the external *perineum-stimulated* anal types and the *motionless* orgasm; not to mention an *imagery-based, Jacuzzi-stimulated,* or *nipple-stimulated* orgasm. Creatively speaking, the list could go on and on based on what is used for stimulation. To say there are exactly ten types, or one hundred types, of orgasms would be pointless.

Nonetheless, some explanation is warranted to interpret the issue. After defining the three major types of orgasms, I'll move to characterizing several obscure subcategories. By way of explanation, I'll then compare each to ice cream, my second favorite thing in the world:

Single means one automatic reflex expressing itself in vaginal contractions, which usually varies in intensity depending on the source of stimulation.

This is like French Vanilla ice cream. It's pure, simple, and delicious.

Multiple refers to more than one orgasm during a single lovemaking session. There's a definite rest period in between climaxing; so it's basically a series of single orgasms with several minutes in between breaking up the tension. Many women require five to ten minutes, or more, to build up to the next one; others need less than two minutes. (According to recent studies, 15 to 25 percent of the population are considered multiorgasmic, although the percentage almost doubles if you consider orally and manually stimulated orgasms.) Typically, multiple orgasms exhibit varying degrees of intensity, often with increasing intensity.

I compare this type to Neapolitan ice cream because the different flavors are represented by a well-defined color.

Sequential is unique. This type is more rare, and, I think, more unpredictable. It's like a stream of orgasms, perhaps six to twelve, one right after another with no break in between. Individually, each orgasm is less intense and less vigorous than a single or multiple, and they also don't last as long. Still, the entire experience is exceptionally fulfilling and physically demanding. It's an incredibly emotional phenomenon.

Like Pistachio Nut, it's very distinctive. The flavor blends together; first you taste the mint, the crunch, then the hazelnut quality.

Additional Types

The *anally stimulated* type includes two categories: 1) The first involves the peritoneal membrane, which lines the abdominal cavity and is reflected inward over the pelvic viscera. Technically, if the stimulation is on the inside of the anus, in the peritoneum area, it should be called a *peritoneal-stimulated* type. 2) If the stimulation occurs on the outside lining, on the perineum, the tissue connecting the anus to the posterior part of the external genitalia, then it should be called a *perineum-stimulated* type. Sometimes the slightest touch of a finger stimulates another orgasm after the initial one.

These words sound so similar, it can be confusing. Both types can be very explosive and give deep, ecstatic pleasure.

> *Regarding the* Perineum *Type, I'd have to go with a triple-decker banana split ice cream. It's almost too much to handle all at once.*

Motionless orgasms can be considered a variation of the sequential or multiple type. Static intercourse is *NOT* going slow or holding back, but rather the result of internal muscle control of the woman. It's the absence of any voluntary intervention. In this case, the man is passive, achieving a state of noneffort. By flexing the inner PC muscle while your partner is perfectly still, a woman's automatic response system takes over, producing unique sequential or multiple orgasms. Until I experienced it myself, I didn't believe self-operating orgasms existed.

Since this type is more difficult to consummate, it shouldn't be the goal of a woman who is striving to achieve regular climaxes. For me, it happens occasionally when the rhythm of intercourse has slowed down to a gentler, magical pace. When my partner is unmistakably hitting my sensitive G-spot, I stop completely as if to signal my intentions. He slows down until becoming totally still. And wow! Because of an involuntary trigger, it's possible to have another five or six orgasms very quickly.

My partner thought it was bizarre the first time it happened. Now it's part of our repertoire. It's a heavenly way to climax, one that causes me to sob tenderly. Once your partner knows you, crying shouldn't trouble him as it might the first time. Explain that your tears are drops of ecstasy. Motionless orgasms make me feel light-headed, as if the blood has rushed out of my mind all at once. This fully relaxed orgasm is more advanced, and once accomplished, produces an overwhelming effect.

How about a hot fudge sundae with a cherry on top?

A Unique Experience

The perineum orgasm gives deep, ecstatic pleasure. The ultimate experience, in my opinion, is a combination of the types listed above. But if you're striving for a unique sensation, try this. Since the perineum is located between the anus and the vagina, a man can stimulate it in several ways. His hand can gently rub the membrane lining on the outside; and his penis can aim for internal stimulation. It requires the deepest penetration possible with the woman on top, or if preferred, in a sitting position.

Remember, the motionless orgasm is more difficult to achieve and considered by many to be the most elusive of all. For me, it's easier to have this type when I'm not trying for it, and it occurs most often after a stream of less intense ones. But some women purposely avoid elaborate foreplay and go straight for deep penetration. In either case, avoid direct manual stimulation of the clitoris. However, any indirect frictional tension around the clitoral shaft caused by the motion of the penis is fine.

If desired, strive for a peritoneal type after a long foreplay session. Try it after a rest period of fifteen to twenty minutes when tension can build again into a high arousal stage. The body needs to be warmed up, perhaps with orally stimulated orgasms. Then, the second time around, arousal culminates quicker in a convulsive climactic shock wave. A peritoneal orgasm is very intense and happens only once. That's why many consider it as an explosive, single type. Motionless orgasms, on the other hand, are usually sequential. Perhaps you're already having them and never attached a name to it.

No matter what I say about these, words fall short of the ecstatic experience. It's like my entire body is electrified, shaking and trembling, stiffening uncontrollably for what seems like a very long time. It's probably only a few minutes in actuality. But, as with most orgasms, time stands still, suspended, turning into a dreamlike eternity.

I feel as if my body has enveloped the universe. I feel light-headed, bordering on a fainting spell, in a limitless dimension of time and space. I am content. I am willing to return to the realities of the day, more aware of being a purposeful individual. I feel mystical and majestic.

Three Stages of Sexual Response

To clear up several other myths and misconceptions about orgasm, let's discuss some technical matters so you have a clear picture of what happens to your body. It's really fascinating what goes on inside our physical temple.

Stage 1—Arousal

Arousal triggers the walls of your vagina to secrete droplets (vaginal lubrication). The amount of moisture depends on several factors:

1) Age
2) Stress
3) Pregnancy
4) Use of tampons
5) Vaginal infections
6) Level of excitement
7) Use of contraceptive pills

It's okay to use a lubricant gel or cream, such as K-Y jelly, if you feel dry. I wouldn't make a big deal about it. Just keep a tube next to your bed, or wherever you make love most often, and keep it within reach. (Incidentally, Vaseline is not water-soluble and therefore is not recommended as a lubricant.) Some women prefer to use a dab of K-Y on their own genitals, while others lubricate their partner's penis prior to penetration. For many couples, it takes away the worry about how well they're lubricated so they're freer to enjoy the experience itself. Nobody should put a guilt trip on the other partner if the female happens to be dry. Why point fingers when there's such an easy solution?

Saliva: A great natural lubricant & always available!

There should be a billboard in everyone's bedroom like this one. Saliva is the greatest natural lubricant. Of course, cunnilingus usually works to lubricate the woman, but it's not always practical. One simple way to insure a smooth and pleasurable penetration is through brief fellatio. Just leave excess dabs of saliva on your mate's penis and an extra bit on the tip. This is fun for both people. Besides, you can signal your readiness this way; his erection already signals his. To tell the truth, I do this virtually every time my partner and I have intercourse for my own sake. If it gives my partner extra pleasure, then so much the better. Personally, I require a graceful entrance into my sacred space. And that's what I get every time.

Also in stage I, your genital area fills with blood, causing the labia (lips) to swell, the clitoris to enlarge, and the clitoral shaft to become erect. As a way to protect itself from this ultrasensitive stage, the clitoris retracts underneath the hood. Trust me, it's still very sensitive there and can be stimulated from indirect pressure.

On the outside, your breasts swell slightly and your nipples stand up erect as well. Some women enjoy only gentle caresses during this phase. On the inside, your uterus enlarges, rising from a resting position. And, finally, your vagina enlarges to accommodate the penis.

Stage II—Plateau

It's called the plateau phase because of a female's ability to stay at a high level of excitement. On the outside, reddish areas appear on your skin which may look like blotches. This occurs due to a change in blood flow and is more noticeable in fair-skinned people. Interestingly, men and women experience similar responses to arousal.

Your breathing and heart rate increase. Your labia minora (inner lips) darken, and your uterus becomes fully elevated, almost balloonlike. Feelings of tension in other parts of your body occur during this state of high sexual excitement. You may experience this as a heaviness in the legs, arms, genitals, and abdomen. It is typically neither pleasant nor unpleasant, but it could be perceived as uncomfortable if you're not accustomed to these feelings. Once you're used to the sensations of arousal, you will learn to appreciate them. Tune in to the experience and enjoy it, even be comforted by these feelings of stimulation. This plateau phase usually leads to the final stage.

Stage III—Orgasmic

This is the reflex itself, which brings a series of rhythmical muscle contractions around the vagina and uterus. Again, each contraction is eight-tenths of a second long, and typically not perceived by the woman as separate contractions. When blood is released in the vaginal lining, you become orgasmic. It's the buildup of body tension via direct or indirect stimulation of the clitoral glans that causes the arousal, which in turn triggers an orgasm. After a sexual release, your body gradually returns to its unaroused state.

Breathing and heart rate decrease, as does the enlargement of breasts, labia, and clitoris. Your uterus goes from a ballooned position to its normal resting position, and your vagina returns to its almost closed normal shape and size. You may even feel revived, ready to run a mile.

Men, on the other hand, generally feel like a nap. This behavior is a chemical reaction, so don't blame them for falling asleep right after sex. It's perfectly natural.

How Similar Is a Man's Orgasm?

The sensation for a man during climax is probably more like a woman's than different. Of course, there's no way to really prove this, but studies show that both sexes produce the same chemicals in the brain, which results in a similar feeling of physiological sensations. The woman's climax typically lasts a little longer than the man's, but the contractions in the body pulsate at the same rate, eight-tenths of a second per contraction. Amazing, but true.

We know that an orgasm is a physical reflex. So what happens exactly? The glans and shaft of the clitoris become swollen (engorged) with blood and expand about thirty times their un-aroused size. Amazingly, the total amount of blood vessel engorgement during arousal can equal or exceed that of a penis.

Did you know that the clitoris is like the tip of a man's penis? In a young fetus, the physical appearance is exactly the same until a certain point in the development, which determines if a boy or girl will be born. The rest of the underlying structure of a female rests internally, of course, but is roughly the same size as the genitalia of a male.

A Woman's Advantage

Personally, I appreciate a woman's advantage. Not only do our orgasms last longer, but, unlike most men, we can have sequential and multiple types. Select gentlemen can climax two or three times in the same night, but this is definitely not the norm. Still, men can't come close to a woman's orgasmic number. With the help of various sources of stimulation, a woman has the potential for scores of orgasms in a single twenty-four hour period. No bragging, just fact. Another wonderful advantage, I think, is that our orgasms can actually become more intense as the stimulation progresses, while a man's are designed to become less intense. Who knows why these physiological discrepancies exist? Just be glad you're a woman. As you can tell, I'm absolutely thrilled.

The Key: Learning to Let Go

An orgasm is a reflex. Simple. It happens when the clitoris is stimulated and a buildup of blood around the vagina is released. So how come you can get aroused and then it fades away? Why do some women have trouble reaching orgasm?

Can you stop a sneeze? Sure. You've probably stifled a sneeze before in a public place because you didn't want to attract attention to yourself. Likewise, you can stifle your own orgasm. Let's look at a few ways women can unintentionally undermine their own pleasure:

- anxious about life
- too much objectivity
- playing a spectator role
- lack of personal involvement
- uptight about sex in general
- stressed about their partner
- worried about getting pregnant

- embarrassed about how they'll act
- embarrassed about how they'll look
- own feelings of guilt for using a man

Obviously it is best to refocus attention on what you feel in your body or on what you feel emotionally in order to experience satisfying orgasms with a partner. Trying too hard will actually hinder your goal, and prevent you from having one.

It's obvious that pain, illness, drugs, alcohol, anxiety, or fatigue affect how you respond sexually. If you've only reached stage II—plateau phase—without ever experiencing an orgasm, you're still normal. But you probably feel very frustrated emotionally and uncomfortable physically from a lack of release. Try not to worry. It's just that you need to learn to let go. Over time, you may have actually learned to shut yourself down sexually to avoid the routine pain and frustration associated with arousal without release. You can overcome this.

Maybe you only desire to be close to a partner without orgasm, and that's okay, too. Men have less of a need for orgasm as they age, a blessing to a woman who needs more time to reach stage III. Many women during the so-called prudish Victorian times had their first orgasm in middle age because their husbands were not as interested in ejaculation as they were in their younger days. Consequently, men kept an erection longer, which allowed the normal rhythmic movements to promote a level of high excitement, leading some women to experience their first orgasm. But not their last!

The important thing is letting go. (More on this in Chapter 9.) Some books recommend that you role-play having an orgasm by yourself even if you actually have never had one, allowing yourself to do whatever you think you would do. Remember, people can respond in different ways each time.

Climaxing is like dancing. You have a certain style, perhaps even a individualistic flair. If you videotaped yourself dancing to various kinds of music, you'd see uniqueness each time. Your patterns of movement would be similar, but you may integrate six or seven styles within a single song. Your dancing is still distinctively you, right?

Like creative tension, two magnets pull between two planets or two dancers. While dancing should be wonderfully exciting, graceful, fun, and loving, there's always the potential for it to be dull, clumsy, unauthentic, or disappointing. In which case, just try again another time. You're not always in the mood for dancing; likewise, you probably aren't always in the mood for sex.

Think of orgasms in the same light. Your pattern of climaxing may vary with your particular mood and energy level. That's okay. In fact, on separate occasions, you may:

- whine
- cry
- talk
- be quiet
- stiffen
- scream
- turn red
- be still
- move erratically
- mumble to yourself
- laugh (if so, prepare your partner)

You may do a combination of these things during one lovemaking session. Let your body and mind guide you. Remember, sexual response is only a matter of time and practice.

Once you have a decent orgasm, it's easier to repeat the experience, and usually in less and less time. Talk about your feelings, fears, and anxieties with your partner ahead of time. If you need an extra nudge to get over the orgasmic hump, try these practical suggestions:

- Breathe purposefully (pant heavily).
- Tense your legs/feet, arms/hands.
- Point your toes and clench your fists.
- Do Kegel exercises (see the next section).
- Lean your head backward to increase blood flow.
- Say erotic words to yourself.
- Say things out loud to your partner, like "yes, yes," "more," or "I want you."
- Tease yourself by lifting away from your partner, slowly meeting again, and get back in sync.
- Try a different pelvic motion from what you do normally.
- Listen to music and get into its rhythms.
- Picture your favorite scenery (or erotic picture).

- Fantasize.
- Tell yourself that you're giving your partner more pleasure than he can endure.

Try to do whatever feels most right and comfortable for your body, your mind, your soul.

Kegel Exercises for Vaginal Muscle Control

Sequential and multiple orgasms work well if the woman has good vaginal muscle control. For those of you who have gone through childbirth classes such as Lamaze, you've already heard of Kegel exercises. A doctor named Arnold Kegel developed the exercise in 1952 to help women with urinary problems. To everyone's delight, the exercises also enhanced genital sensation and increased the likelihood for orgasms.

Two easy exercises are the following:

1—Midflow exercise.
2—Elevator exercise.

1) There's a muscle that helps control the flow of urine that all women are familiar with, even if we don't know it by name. It's called the pubococcygeal muscle (PC muscle for short). During urination, try to stop and start your flow three, four, or five times. Do this with your legs fairly well apart. Then empty your bladder well. (It's not good to do this too often without completely emptying the bladder.)

Once you know the exact feel of this muscle, you can practice this without urinating. Before my first child was born, I used to practice at stoplights or in the office when I was talking to someone I didn't particularly like. It made me feel good. I could sit there and do Kegels, and they were too stupid to notice. Of course, nobody could ever tell you're doing an internal exercise.

2) Next, advance to the elevator exercise. Here, you use the same muscle and pretend to start at the bottom of an elevator and slowly squeeze as you go up. Once at the top, you come back down. The best way to see if you can do this is to ask your partner if he can feel you squeezing. Then, ask him to tell you when he can't feel the pressure any longer. The first few times he may just feel pressure on the first

level. Later, he may be able to discern three or four levels, or more.

It's almost a guarantee that your sex life will improve if you're willing to try these simple exercises.

Women, listen up! You never need to complain about being stuck in traffic or waiting for the light to change. Seize the opportunity to do Kegels! Think about it. You're improving your chances for having orgasms every time you exercise your PC muscle. Never waste time in traffic again! When I'm stopped at a red light, I frequently begin my Kegels. Like Pavlov's dogs, it's become an automatic response. It works for me. It can do wonders for you, too!

6

Other Common Myths & Misconceptions

In the last chapter, we covered just about everything you wanted to know about orgasm and weren't afraid to ask. Now let's talk about four additional misconceptions. As we discuss these myths, the one important distinction that can free us from the hold of memories of past misrepresentations is to move from left-brain to right-brain thinking. As a reminder, the right side synthesizes experiences creatively while the left hemisphere correlates to the analytical.

Ask yourself, "Am I making love or just having sex?" Like the difference between writing and editing, one is the creative process, and the other is necessary to perfect the job. Having sex is a learned behavior. It relies on techniques we've learned and applied to another human being. This works, but it's mechanical. If you're afraid you'll make a mistake, look or feel silly, or forget the so-called right technique, then nothing enchanted happens. Sex becomes automated. Like revising faulty grammar, *having sex* is the "correct and perfect" method where two people say things like "put your hand here, do this, faster, slower, more tender please." Periodically a couple may need to refine their encounters, but eventually they move on to resourceful, inventive sex with love. *Making love* is the free release of emotions that lets *spirited sex* happen. When you focus on the act of loving instead of technique, something unexpected happens. Something magical.

With that in mind, we're going to cover ways to use right-brain thinking about other common misconceptions. This chapter highlights two fallacious myths:

1) That the ultimate experience is the simultaneous orgasm.
2) That self-pleasure is a naughty, unhealthy activity.

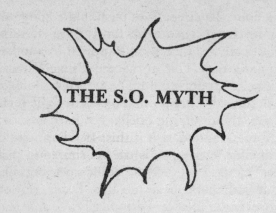

THE S.O. MYTH

The Myth Surrounding Simultaneous Orgasm

Simultaneous orgasm refers to both individuals climaxing at the exact same time. It does happen. That part is not a myth. Some people view it as the ultimate proof of true love. In my mind, however, it's the ultimate proof of a lucky coincidence. (Even an Arabian camel finds a water hole in the desert once in a while!)

If you have this expectation, you may be sorely disappointed when it doesn't occur. And unless you have sex down to a science, which it's not, then you're bound to be frustrated much of the time. Don't get me wrong, simultaneous orgasms can happen more often with some couples than others, but it's not likely to occur on a regular basis. Human beings are not programmable machines, ready at the flick of a button to perform functions at will.

The way I look at it is this: If it happens, it does. If it doesn't, so what? As simple as that sounds, I believe it to be a healthy attitude. In my opinion, it's ridiculous to perpetually try for simultaneous orgasms. Every now and then, a couple may want to spice up the encounter and go for it. But typically, it puts an unrealistic pressure on both partners to perform, lessening the enjoyment of the sexual sensations at the time.

Can you imagine the dialogue that goes on between a couple trying too hard for a simultaneous orgasm?

John says, "I'm almost there."
"But I'm not ready," Carol responds.
"Hurry up, sweetheart."
"I'm going as fast as I can."
"Oh, please," John implores.
"Slow down, wait for me."
"I can't wait any longer."

Carol begs, "Hold back just a minute."

"A minute?" he asks incredulously.

"I'm not quite ready..."

Unable to hold back any longer, John declares, "I'm about to come!"

"Wait, I'm not there yet!" she shrieks.

"Aaaaaaaaaaaaaaaah!"

"You SOB!" she says angrily. "I didn't come yet."

"Sorry, honey, I couldn't help it," he says. "Keep trying, I've still got some left in me."

"Thanks, but no thanks," Carol sulks.

John and Carol have not made love. They've participated in a sexual circus. Like the guy who spins fifteen plates on top of sticks at the same time, it's hard to do. Perfect timing is required. If one plate stops spinning, frustration results. Likewise, when partners try too hard for simultaneous orgasms, resentment can set in. It's not worth it.

Believe me, I'm not trying to downplay the emotional satisfaction of simultaneous orgasm. Personally, I think it's splendid when it happens. In fact, women who have orgasms throughout a sexual encounter are more likely to experience it. More important, however, is not to put pressure on your partner.

First the man should make sure the woman

is satisfied. There's no reason to insist on exact timing. When a man is ready to climax, fine. In this way, he can enjoy his orgasm more fully. He's been a gentleman and now deserves to come when he wants. His mate may come again when he's climaxing, but it's not paramount for her fulfillment.

Still, simultaneous orgasm is not my idea of the ultimate sexual experience. Having separate orgasms has its own advantages. For a woman, she can have as many as she has the energy for, allowing her partner to appreciate her orgasmic expression more fully without the distraction of his own orgasm. For a man to feel your excitement building, to hear your sounds, to be close to you emotionally during your orgasm, is a special experience with its own reward.

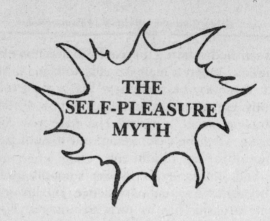

THE SELF-PLEASURE MYTH

The Joy of Self-Pleasure

Self-pleasure can be a normal, healthy part of life. Most folks today realize you won't go blind or grow hair on the palms of your hands if you masturbate. Still, I think many misconceptions exist about the subject. Usually it's at its height during one's teens or during periods of loneliness and stress in adulthood. For many, masturbation is no longer a dirty word in our society, and rightly so. According to one study, 85 percent of the population have masturbated at some time in their lives. The remaining group, those who don't engage, miss out on a totally natural experience. If it were wicked, why would innocent babies and toddlers do it?

Clearly, a majority of women masturbate on a regular basis. You need to know what pleases you before being pleased by a partner. Of course, you can discover this with the help of a man, but it takes a rare mate to guide you through this trial-and-error method. Think of the pitfalls in telling a man what he's doing does not please you. If you tried something on yourself, you might say, "Okay, that didn't work; I'd better go on with something else." But can you imagine the ego and pride involved in telling your partner, "Honey, try something different because that didn't feel so good"? Even the most tactful person in the world is likely to cause hurt feelings. Worse still, your partner may not want to try something new and adventurous for fear of being rejected in the future. You both lose out.

In all fairness, I want to write about the potential negative side of masturbation. Only two kinds of harm could come from it: 1) physical harm from too much friction or use of unclean objects, and 2) emotional harm if the person's moral, religious, or psychological background creates so much guilt, it becomes traumatic, where the benefits do not outweigh the drawbacks. Of course, these two upsets could also happen from manual manipulation with a partner or from intercourse itself.

I know several women who have suffered tremendous amount of guilt over masturbating until they finally made a deliberate choice to separate themselves from outmoded messages handed down to them as children. A few friends needed outside professional services to rid themselves of this ingrained guilt. Now they're delighted with the results of the consultation and their newfound freedom.

The Advantages of Self-Enjoyment

The advantages outweigh the disadvantages. If you stop and think about it, masturbation is:

- simple
- effective
- available
- legal
- safe
- pregnancy-proof

It also has other positive features. Self-pleasure:

- adds variety to life
- improves mental health
- enriches private fantasies

- leads to understanding self
- helps during stressful phases
- assists during periods of loneliness
- does not require emotional attachment
- releases tension without performance worry
- requires less physical energy than intercourse
- helps women focus energy to reach personal goals

With reasons like these, who needs intercourse anyway? (Just kidding!) Most important, women who see masturbation as an essential part of body awareness are well on the road to easier, dependable orgasms.

Suggested Equipment: Buy a Vibrator

I used to think that a vibrator was superficial. I'd prided myself on being a natural sort of person. As a gag gift for Christmas one year, I was given an electric vibrator with seven attachments. Much later, I discovered it was no joke and overcame my hesitation about using a so-called superficial method. It was simple and much more efficient. On particularly horny days, I found myself using it several times.

Basically, I use it once or twice a week, or whenever the mood strikes. After a few orgasms, I can think more clearly and accomplish my day's goals without being consumed with the need for a sexual release. Otherwise, I lack focus. Have you ever felt like that?

We take for granted many electrical devices to help us enhance the quality of our lives. For example, we may use a toaster, an electric shaver, an alarm clock, a flashlight, a coffeepot, a hair blower, and a washer and dryer regularly. In the sexual area, however, a vibrator is considered unnatural, abnormal, or a crutch by many people. How is it more of a crutch than an alarm clock to help us get out of bed in the morning? Often the idea of what is right comes from what we learned as a child, what we picked up from our specific background. Rethink those antiquated messages and decide for yourself.

Think of a vibrator as a tool, like any other device we use for convenience and efficiency. It's something that makes life easier. You can go to any department store and ask for a massager without any embarrassment. If you don't mind telling a fib, just say you need something to relax sore muscles after playing tennis. In major cities, many lingerie stores carry vibrators for sexually explicit purposes. Compare models and buy a well-built, safe, light one that suits you. Buy one with various attachments, if that intrigues you, or try the dildo type if you prefer. (I've gotten *attached* to the external type myself.)

Of course, the experience of masturbating can be pleasant no matter what you use for stimulation. But it's likely to be longer-lasting and more intense with a vibrator. To add icing to the cake, you can reach orgasm quicker because you have total control over the situation.

The point is, a woman deserves to have a physical release without the constraints and demands of having a man to fulfill her desires. Besides, are you always in the mood for companionship, conversation, romance, dinner, or diplomacy?

If not, you're simply treating your man like an object if you want him to participate in your physical release. Now, tell the truth; won't you be a little resentful if you ask and he's not in the mood? While that's a natural reaction when your hormones are going crazy, it's silly when you have a simple, workable option.

Anyway, masturbation is so much more efficient. Of course, it lacks the personalized, emotional side of sex, but that's not what we need every time. And the reality of modern times is that most women go without a sex partner for long periods due to temporary impotence, divorce, separation, widowhood, or by choice. Even being married is no guarantee that you're getting enough sex.

For most of us, our mental health rests partly on the physical release of sexual tension. What's perfect about the vibrator is that one can vary the speed by the push of a button. I usually start out on the low speed as a warm-up and move it to the high speed whenever I'm ready for the "kick." You can also vary the pitch or angle and pressure for a unique set of sensations.

Women can become comfortable with the idea of experimenting with their vibrators. After psychological barriers are broken down, a woman can experience as many orgasms as she's willing to take. In the beginning, I used to build up to one "big" climax and think I was finished. It took months of dedicated practice, but eventually I discovered how to satiate myself with as many as two dozen orgasms. I'm a glutton for satisfaction. When separated from my partner, though, I never feel desperate or needy. That's good news! Successful masturbation may even decrease women's desire for meaningless affairs just because they're horny. Consequently, men should encourage their mates to buy a vibrator rather than feel threatened.

Think of self-pleasure as a learning process for climaxing with a partner. Try not to miss out on a remarkable, easy opportunity to know your own body. You, too, can become comfortable with the idea of experimenting with a vibrator. Believe me, don't knock it until you've dared to experiment.

After all, who knows best when, where, how much, how fast, or how slow you want it!

The Magic of Masturbation

Be aware of how your breathing rhythms quicken during masturbation. You'll be able to relax and come with your sex partner more easily once you know the signs. Sometimes let your body stiffen up while climaxing, a natural reaction under the circumstances. In gaining more control, you can also learn how to relax through a less intense orgasm. This adds a different dimension to the sensation. While purposely building up to an intense orgasm, bring your body to near-climax about five or six times before concentrating directly on the clitoris.

When ready, position yourself for an intense orgasm that stiffens your body for as long as a minute. (Relatively speaking, this *is* a long time.) If you decide to relax your body, you may feel more like you're on clouds, a magical floating sensation, which can last a lot longer than a minute. And if you mix the two, you may be able to go ten or fifteen minutes before stopping. (My vibrator overheats by then anyway!)

For many years, I wasn't comfortable with the idea of touching my breasts during masturbation. But why do we think it's strange to touch our chest when we're going to touch our vaginal area? From a strictly logical point of view, it doesn't make any sense. I'm sure the way we are raised has a lot to do with how we view the entire subject. Have you found that touching your breasts during the warm-up stage enhances the experience? By pairing the sensation of nipple stimulation with orgasm, it will more likely repeat itself when done with a partner. This is called "anchoring." That's when one intense experience is associated so strongly that it triggers another response. More on that subject in Chapter 8.

Self-Pleasure Leads to Better Sex

Haven't you always wondered how the experts study masturbation? They interview, take surveys, or observe and record physical reactions. The common thread among research was this: Masturbation is an individual matter of choice and preference. There were several common beliefs and suggestions, however, that warrant repeating.

Most of the research I've read concludes that women who masturbate are more likely to be orgasmic, that it enhances their sexual desire with a partner. So if you fear getting self-obsessed, don't worry. You'll probably enjoy sex more after experimenting with masturbation.

Sex therapists generally tell clients to try different strokes, different ways of touching. First the outer lips, moving to the inner lips, then to the shaft, hood, and head of the clitoris. Circular motions seemed to be the most common, although gentle up and down pressures also were found effective. Rocking the pelvis in the same thrusting motions as during intercourse on top of objects or directly on top of the bed were used frequently as well.

Vary the rhythm, strokes, and pressure

when you are first learning to give pleasure to yourself. Use a lubricant such as K-Y jelly or another water-soluble cream or gel (not Vaseline). Your natural secretions will vary with the time of day, place, and amount of time spent in arousal.

In short, think of self-pleasure as a learning process for climaxing with a partner. You'll recognize the unique signs of buildup and how it feels just prior to release. Once you know how your body responds, you'll be better able to trigger that same response with your lover. In this manner, you can cultivate a capacity for more orgasms during intercourse if you want.

The Continuum of Emotions

Overall, does masturbation bring up positive or negative feelings for you? Although this is hopefully changing, many women feel guilty, foolish, lonely, uncomfortable, ashamed, self-conscious, and generally negative about the experience. Others sum it up by saying, "Physically, it feels good; psychologically, I feel empty."

Obviously, our associations of loneliness, rejection, childhood punishment, or social pressure influence the way we feel. But we can try to overcome negative feelings by substituting more rational statements for nonrational tapes that play in our head. Why do women think that an orgasm is more valuable when they are with a man? Do we really have to please a man in order to feel precious? I think not. During periods of stress, loneliness, or separation from a mate, you have the freedom to masturbate more frequently. Even if you're married or have a steady man in your life, it doesn't mean you should automatically stop. Quit if you like, but it's not necessary. In fact, I believe it'll significantly improve your sex life together.

Again, masturbation is a normal and healthy outlet. If you think it's a lonely business, it will be. But so is making love to a person who doesn't love or care for you in return. Another irrational statement is one you may have heard as a child by older kids on the block: If you play with yourself, you're emotionally incomplete. Actually, masturbation can help us keep an emotional balance because we are free from the ache or desire that goes along with a lack of sexual release. This is especially true if we're used to a sexual outlet with a partner and he is suddenly taken away from us through a temporary or permanent situation: extended travel, illness, disability, impotency, separation, divorce, or death.

Other women have only positive feelings associated with masturbation. Besides the fact that the orgasms are very intense and numerous, many feel they deserve to treat themselves. Remember, you have the right to please yourself. Enjoy the experience both physically and psychologically. Hooray!

As you can see, there's a wide range of emotions and viewpoints on the subject. Feelings vary from complete enjoyment, to satisfied, but guilty (or some other negative emotion), to dissatisfaction, or total avoidance. Try to evaluate why you feel the way you do. Only you can decide what's best for you in the long run, but keep an open mind. Let your body and heart be your guide!

7

Is There Sex After Motherhood?

Nobody likes to be stereotyped. Mothers and seasoned citizens are no exception. Consequently, this chapter highlights two additional erroneous myths:

1) Motherhood and *spirited sex* don't mix.
2) The aging process prevents good sex.

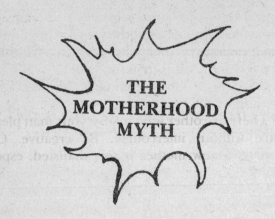

THE
MOTHERHOOD
MYTH

Motherhood and Spirited Sex

There seems to be a nagging myth that motherhood and *spirited sex* just don't mix. Well, I'm here to tell you that's wrong. Misconceptions like this get started by stereotyping people. Several men have told me that their wives just weren't interested in sex after having babies. My first question to them is: "How soon after childbirth did you expect to have sex with your wife?" closely followed by, "How have you treated your wife since the birth of your child?"

Granted, some women heal faster than others; but I wish men could have children so they'd be a little more sensitive to the miraculous hell a woman's body goes through during pregnancy, labor, and delivery. We may not feel like intercourse for several weeks afterward. My doctor recommends six weeks of healing before having sex.

There are other ways to give your man pleasure without intercourse. Be creative. Of course, a new mother is so exhausted, especially those first three weeks, that she's typically NOT interested in sex. What a small price to pay for such a precious human being in your life! Let's say your man is very patient and considerate; still, explain to him that you may have to go slow in the beginning to get back into the swing of things. Don't expect a night of passionate lovemaking just because you've waited five or six weeks. Sometimes this happens, but most likely, it takes time to readjust your attitude as well as your body. As we discussed in Chapter 4, good sex is 90 percent mental.

A woman doesn't want to feel like a vehicle for his desires; yet, understandably, a man may be frustrated by a lack of sex. Of course, happily, he can masturbate during this period. The best thing a man can do to get their sex life back on track is to make his partner feel special out of bed. More important, he needs to reinforce his mate's sense of womanhood through her sexual identity as well as her role as a mother. If he's not very creative about stuff like this or needs suggestions, tell him specifically what he could do to make you feel more loving, or simply give him the following list:

- Offer a "free" night of massaging her feet, back, arms, legs, etc.

- Have a glass of special hot tea or a glass of wine together.

- Take a hot bath together with candles all around the tub.

- Go to the movies again like you used to in the preparenthood days.

- Send fresh flowers or a card to celebrate her "unbirthday."

- Encourage her to visit friends while you take care of the baby.

- Take her to that special place you both like so well.

- Write a provocative note and tell her how special she is.

- Cook a simple dinner or clean the house.

Well, this is a good start. When there's true love in a relationship, a previously active female will get back into the sexual swing of things after having children. Trust me, I think sex gets even better after having kids. A woman may feel more personally fulfilled if she's wanted kids for a long time. She may be more at peace with herself and the world, perhaps. For me, there was an improvement after having children. Undoubtedly other factors enter into the equation; but all in all, it gets better. Much better.

Physical Realities After Childbirth

Physically speaking, a woman can get back into shape within one year after giving birth. There are few legitimate reasons why women keep on the previous weight gain after that point. So some ladies need encouragement to have a regular exercise routine, join a health club, or visit a nutritionist. Perhaps you can start a new pattern of walking or riding bikes as a couple. Take the baby with you until you can get a reliable and affordable baby-sitter.

Many women are concerned that their vag-

childbirth. On the positive side, the vagina usually reverts to the same size it was originally. If you believe there's been a physical change or if there's pain associated with intercourse after childbirth, you need to consult your gynecologist. If your doctor says it's all in your mind, get a second or even a third opinion. There have been rare cases where some doctors were not capable of diagnosing the problem; and in a small percentage of cases, minor surgery was required to fix the situation.

I emphasize *rare*. Even after having numerous children, the shape of a woman's vagina changes very little. I've been assured by one man that even though his wife feels marginally less taut than before, the sex is just as good. Perhaps the angle of penetration needs to be adjusted, that's all. If you're concerned, refer to Chapter 5 for exercises that help tone up an internal vaginal muscle called the pubococcygeal muscle (PC for short), and consult your gynecologist. Remember the PC muscle works like any other in your body; use it or lose its effectiveness. The more you exercise it, the stronger it gets, and the greater your chances for climaxing easily.

Only Mothers Know for Sure

Here are a few representative samples of women's comments about the Motherhood Myth:

- "Our kids are teenagers now, and they're never home. So we've found more time on our hands—it's been great rediscovering each other."

- "It's harder to find the time these days. I miss the closeness."

- "I can't explain it, but I wasn't the least bit interested in sex for about five months after Amy was born ... By then, my husband seemed preoccupied. We're discussing how to get back on track right now. That's why I came to your seminar."

- "Unfortunately, it took a tragedy in our lives to make us appreciate how special our sex was to us. Now we actually schedule time regularly; we haven't given up spontaneous sex, but it doesn't happen as often as it did before our kids were born. It's still beautiful."

- "My husband wanted it five days after Matt was born; we just never seemed to miss a beat. I was pretty tired...but he didn't seem to mind."

• "Less than a year after our second child arrived, my husband left me. I was devastated. After that, I was celibate for almost two years and didn't miss sex one bit. But a few months ago, I met a wonderful man, and now I'm enjoying sex again. It's better now than it ever was with my husband."

In brief, good sex and motherhood can coexist splendidly. Remember that good sex is 90 percent mental. So keep in mind this slight twist of a famous line by Abraham Lincoln: *Most folks are as sexual as they make up their minds to be.*

THE AGING MYTH

The misconception that aging hinders good sex stems from several issues. Traditionally the United States has been a youth-oriented society. This is now changing, primarily because of the baby-boomer power base (those born between 1946 and 1964). The last batch of this population will reach middle age in the nineties. The conventional older generation was brought up not to discuss the subject of sex privately, much less publicly. Consequently, how do we determine if they have a quality sex life? Most pollsters don't even ask the question.

The longer one lives, obviously, the greater the chance for disability, illness, and accidents to take their natural toll. Also, one's energy level generally decreases as we age. These factors could interfere with one's sex life, but not necessarily. A fifty-seven-year-old friend recently disclosed that he and his girlfriend make love nearly every day, and sometimes twice a day on weekends. Besides, energetic older folks have more time on their hands to enjoy sex if they so choose.

The most important fact to be aware of is that people can have sex at any age, perfectly healthy or not. It's an individual choice and preference. What's old to one person is young to another, so even this myth is rather subjective. To someone in her early twenties, a thirty-five-year-old woman is *old*. To a sixty-seven-year-old, she's young.

Recently I asked my lively septuagenarian mother how old her friend was, and she responded, "Oh, he's young ... I'd say he's about my age." Chuckling, I asked, "Mom, then what's *old* to you?" "Fifteen years older than I am," she said without missing a beat. Youth is definitely in the eye of the beholder. With an attitude like that, my mom is going to stay young at heart for the rest of her life.

What to Look Forward To (Unless You're Already There)

Recent studies have shown some good news for a change. They indicate the possibility for a continuous good sex life if you desire it. There are logical and physiological reasons for this encouraging news.

- Most middle-age women are emotionally stable and at peace with themselves. This allows them to fully express their love and affection to another person. Evidently, anxiety decreases testosterone. So it makes sense that a calm, mature woman would be more responsive than a nervous greenhorn.

- As a woman ages, her estrogen level decreases while her testosterone level stays the same. If you recall, testosterone is responsible for sex drive.

- Some women over forty, especially after childbirth, experience a biological benefit in the form of a weakening of their clitoral tissues. As the walls of the clitoris relax, there is easier access to it. Consequently, less friction causes even greater excitement in many women. Others claim the vein system around the genitals enlarges, which increases sexual exhilaration for an older woman.

Many women over forty-five tell me they crave sex more now than when they were younger. Simply put, they want the carnal gratification and emotional bonding it delivers. More good news: Older women claim their same-age partners want the intimacy and closeness as well. Thankfully, a man's focus can change as he ages. Numerous men are motivated by love and a sense of familiarity rather than just pure physical pleasure.

A mature couple can discover provocative seduction and a newfound playfulness in bed because they don't have to pretend to be all grown-up. They are. Since they don't have to act mature, they can act like kids again—except they're armed with a host of erotic experiences. Who says there's nothing to look forward to when we're older?

Put These Myths Behind You, Where They Belong

Real love means having the freedom to explore sexual adventures of passion. Don't be dictated to by past experiences, myths, and misconceptions. To sum up, say good-bye to these myths. Say hello to "right-brain thinking" and realize: 1) separate orgasms have merits and advantages; 2) self-pleasure is healthy and practical in today's world; 3) sex can actually improve after childbirth; and 4) older people are sexual beings with the time and potential for good sex.

We must also change our thinking and welcome all nuances of lovemaking, even the so-called downtime when your man is trying to get inspired. When we don't insist on technique, we can then experience sex as a creative act of expressive love.

I've come to the conclusion that good lovers are **NOT** special, extratalented, or more sensitive than the average person. Good lovers are simply two people engaged in a sustained and natural extension of survival skills we all have. Moreover, their sexual creations are brought on by the trust in stray impulses to find satisfying patterns.

> *Give up myths about sex and free yourself to do something special: Express a profound, spiritual love to your mate!*

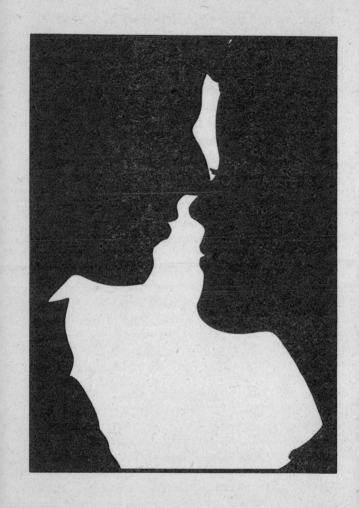

8

Getting Your Partner to Meet Your Needs

As in most things, communication is the key to success. Good fortune in bed is no different. There, talking is no less necessary than other modes of communication, although touching is probably the simplest and most profound way to communicate with another human. The potential for variety adds to the possibility for satisfying results. If words don't come easily to you, you can try other ways to make your point. Moving your partner's hand to where you want it, for example, or simply moaning pleasantly, usually gets a repeat performance.

It's a shame there aren't more assertive women who could have super sex if they could only spit out the words "slower," "faster," or "can you move one half millimeter to the left, please?" A simple request, stated lovingly, will surely be received in that light: "Do that again, but softer" or "I love it when you kiss me rough." Besides, what's a moment of embarrassment compared to a better sex life?

The Dos and Don'ts of Bedroom Communication

DOs:

1. *Be Specific.* How can your partner repeat the behavior if he's not exactly sure what it is you like? During the afterglow, say, "I love the way you lick my earlobe" or "I go crazy when you bite my buns."

2. *Be Generous.* Frequently, but not obsequiously, compliment your mate's good points. Make him feel like he's number one in your book! Hopefully this comes naturally, so it's not forced.

3. *Be Honest.* Emotional dishonesty only leads to feelings of resentment or anger in the long run. A sweetly worded re-

quest will most likely be taken the right way. Being honest is NOT rudeness.

4. *Be Positive.* When making a request for a change in behavior, use positive phrasing. Instead of "Don't rush me," say, "Let's go slower, please." Use an I-message like "I'm feeling a little rushed right now," or, better yet, "I like it when you take your time."

DON'Ts:

1. *Don't Talk in the Bedroom.* Don't discuss any problems in the bedroom, especially sexual ones. Do it eyeball to eyeball at the kitchen table or in another neutral spot. Reserve the bedroom for sleeping, reading, relaxing, or lovemaking. You anchor positive feelings there.

2. *Don't Be Distasteful* Don't start a request with negative, vulgar, or babyish talk such as "you never do as much for me as I do for you," or "You SOB, I hate that," or "Come on, tootsie wootsie, tell Mama all about it." (Whatever you find distasteful should be out in the open. Each couple must decide for themselves, of course.)

3. *Don't Bombard.* Don't tell him he needs to improve in a dozen areas—sexual or otherwise. That'll overwhelm him, or worse, demotivate him. Take one or two issues at a time and resolve them. Reinforce these before moving to the next item. One every sixty days may be the best approach in the beginning.

4. *Don't Nag.* It's difficult to define nagging, but I suspect we intuitively know when it's happening (no matter what end we're on). My guideline is: Don't bring up the same subject more than two to three times per month. These things take time to sink in.

Whether you've been with your partner for twenty days or twenty years, I can't overemphasize the importance of praising his talent. Then you're in a better position to ask for more of a particular delight. Don't flood him with ten requests at the same time; he'll panic! Don't say he's a good kisser if he's not. Find something you especially like. If you can't find one single thing to praise your mate about, I suggest you reconsider why you're with him in the first place.

Variety, skill, and endurance are nice, but

not to the point where sexual athletics and prowess are more important than the love-making itself. Men who need to prove themselves by outperforming other men in bed do not make the best partners either. Unwittingly, many men think they're God's gift to women simply because they can keep it up for an hour. Granted a long-standing erect penis is helpful, but that feat alone does not a good lover make.

The Worth Is in the Girth

Some men pride themselves on size. This old expression sums it up more accurately: *"It's not the size of the boat, but the motion of the ocean that counts."* In regard to dimension, it's the width of a penis, not the length so often joked about, that matters most. The worth is in the man's girth, if anything. Seriously, a wide penis is more likely to create the necessary friction on the clitoris that is mandatory for most orgasms; as a penis moves in the vagina, the extra thickness creates more pressure, which, in turn, stimulates the hood and shaft of a woman's most sensitive area.

Have you ever made love to a man who was so well endowed that you actually had second thoughts about going to bed with him? Believe it or not, an oversize penis can hinder pleasure for a woman unless he takes particular time to lubricate her properly and penetrate slowly. Most women can adapt to such a man, of course, and enjoy the results of nature's accidental blessing. By the way, an unstretched vagina is four inches long, but it's very elastic. Most women can accommodate the man no matter what size he is.

Remember never to comment negatively about the size of a man's penis. Think how hurt you would be if a man criticized the size of your breasts, even though you know that has absolutely nothing to do with sexiness or how stimulated you can be. The truth of the matter is that serviceability of a penis has nothing to do with size. The average erect penis is six inches long. Incidentally, don't comment on how big it is if it's not—your man has undoubtedly measured his. (Still, I'd take girth over length anytime.)

Relatively speaking, a short penis can touch the sensitive nerves of a woman's vagina. Approximately 90 percent of all nerve fibers are located in the first third of your vagina. Remember, thickness matters more; so if his width is plentiful enough and his pelvic thrusts are anatomically placed, the clitoris will be stimulated. The woman can determine the angle of this motion. (More about positions in Chapter 9.) Positioning and magnitude definitely contribute to having multiple orgasms if so desired.

Differences Between the Sexes

A man's sexual response is usually triggered by visual things like your hair, breasts, buttocks, or clothes. Don't be confused by this. These things excite him, allowing him to express his love and affection and desire for you. A man's response is typically, but not always, brisker than a woman's. Women generally make love with their heart. Things may be less important to her, although many women claim to get excited by their men wearing sexy underwear or clothing. Female turn-ons usually involve atmosphere, mood, and how sentimentally attached she is to her mate.

Women need to understand another basic thing about men. Most male sexual feelings are centered in the last inch of the penis. This explains, partially, why most men are so genitally centered. That's why they may play with your genitals before you're ready. Just say, "Honey, could you kiss me a little more first? I love it when you do that."

Touching a penis usually gets your mate in the mood for intercourse fast, so time this carefully with what you want. If you go full bore ahead, he'll want you right away. Go slow, if that's what you want, stroking his penis only occasionally until you're heated up and ready for him to penetrate you.

The Reality of Matching Appetites

Sometimes I wonder if anyone is perfectly happy with the amount of sex they're getting, unless it's in the early stages of a relationship. Both males and females complain about matching appetites, which reminds me of a scene from one of Woody Allen's best movies, *Annie Hall.* Woody is at his therapist's office (where else?), complaining that his girlfriend hardly ever has sex with him—"We only have sex three times a week." In Diane Keaton's scene with the therapist, she sees it differently: "He wants it constantly—three times a week."

What is the norm? I've heard reports of anywhere from 1 to 2.5 times a week. In the fall of 1991, one study revealed these statistics:

Married couples average 67 times per year (1.2 times per week)

Divorced people average 55 times per year (1.0 times per week)

Widowed people average 6 time per year (once every 2 months)

[No statistics on "never-been-married" singles]

The women in my seminars express a wide range of desires. On the low end are those perfectly content with having sex two to three times per month. A few enjoy it almost daily. The "norm" seems to be about twice a week.

The most shocking information from this study, however, was the average length of the lovemaking session itself. Would you believe 12½ minutes? (That's a "swift quickie" in my book!) While I've never done a mathematical analysis, many women tell me they usually spend around thirty minutes in bed with their partner. From beginning to end. So perhaps the 12½ minutes refers to penetration only. Who knows where some of these statistics come from? Statistics are not important anyway (unless a woman feels cheated and wants more, yet hasn't the personal experience to verify what else is available.) A woman needs to know the difference between a realistic expectation and false hope. One is caviar, the other is anchovies.

If You're Getting Less Sex than You Want

Several books have come out specializing in ISD and LSD—inhibited sex desire and limited sex drive. Basically, they're the same thing. Whether physical or psychological, it's real. Men and women should be checked out physiologically first if the lack of sex is causing severe problems in a relationship. Psychological causes may be more difficult to pin down and take longer to remedy, but it's worth the effort for a precious connection.

If you're getting less sex, chances are it's related to one of these issues:

1) Time Allocation—job schedules, kids, stress, community obligations, etc.

2) Health Issues—lack of energy and well-being or the presence of pain.

3) Anger—one person feels the need to control, and chooses sex as a weapon.

4) Low Self-esteem—one partner is disappointed in him or herself; perhaps a job, a large sum of money, or status in the community has been lost.

5) Fear of Intimacy could stem from a childhood fear of abandonment.

6) Third Party Involved—someone is having an affair and channeling sexual energy and affection to another person.

Granted some of these issues are easier to deal with than others, but that's the reality of our society. Consider your situation and then try to make a rational plan and solve the dilemma.

If you're unhappy now, what can you do to increase or decrease your current sexual activity level? Is there a healthy way to compromise?

Of course. Besides encouraging both parties to have physical checkups, I recommend talking to your partner in a straightforward manner using positive terms. Then reinforce any effort made toward your mutual goal. Let's say the man wants sex six or seven times a week, while the woman honestly wants it twice a week. They could compromise on three or four times a week. Then they could decide some of the details ahead of time. A loving couple anticipates problems and resolves them before the situation escalates. One solution might include these elements: who initiates, what time is best to approach, how long some sessions will be, how to say no so it sounds like a postponement instead of a rejection.

If one person insists on sex or humiliates his or her mate when the other declines, it's probably a sign of a sex addict. It's primarily an issue of control, not sexual urges (although some folks simply have very high sexual appetites). This is beyond the scope of this book. So if this sounds familiar, I suggest you seek the professional advice of a marriage/sex counselor immediately. Women married at a young age may never realize what it's like to be in a healthy sexual relationship until after they're divorced. Now in their forties, they may be enjoying sex again because of a caring, balanced partner.

Do You Know What You Really Want?

Surprisingly, most women agree that it's easier to have sex than to talk about it. Even those who are assertive and feel comfortable communicating in bed may not really know exactly what it is they do want. Some woman say, "I just want to feel closer to my partner." Or "It's the same ol' thing week after week." That's not very specific, is it? What's a man going to do with a comment like that? Not much, and I don't blame him. We'll discuss how to communicate your needs in a nonthreatening way to get the results you deserve.

But, first, fill in the blanks so you'll get a clearer picture of what you want:

1. My partner knows I'm ready to be penetrated because _____

   _____

2. When I get very excited, sometimes my partner inadvertently interferes with my orgasm by _____

   _____

3. Lubrication is something I _____

   _____

4. When my partner feels my breasts, I usually _____

   _____

5. I wish I knew more about _____

   _____

6. My favorite stimulation to achieve orgasm is _____

   _____

7. When I perform oral sex on my partner, I feel _____

   _____

8. I wish my partner had better technique when it comes to _____

_____

9. When my partner performs oral sex on me, I usually _____

_____

10. I know I excite my partner when

_____

_____

You, and only you, can decide what you want from a sexual encounter with your mate. To be fulfilled, you have to be honest with yourself. From that point on, you're free to use whatever tools you're comfortable with. Remember, your sincerity and enthusiasm go a long way toward making a companionship work. Perhaps one idea suggested here grabs you more than the others. That's fine. Go with it.

The Power of Positive Reinforcement

Let's assume you are in a balanced relationship. Positive reinforcement is the most basic, yet effective, way to get more of what you want.

What is it? Simply put, positive reinforcement is whatever increases the desired behavior. What works for one person could be agonizing to another. So the trial-and-error method is the right approach. Of course, sincerity is equally important. Reinforcers essentially come in two flavors: tangible and nontangible. Remember primary and secondary reinforcers from Psych 101? Well, forget all that. Just concentrate on what works. Whether you want traditional, off-the-wall, or downright kinky, here's a list of ways to reinforce the special man in your life:

Verbal ways:

- "Oh, yes, oh God, yes, yes . . ."
- "Don't stop, don't stop."
- "You're incredible!"
- "You make me so happy when you . . ."
- "You have magic fingers."
- "I love the way you lick my arms."
- "You make me feel so womanly."
- "Ride 'em, cowboy . . . giddyap, little dogie."

- "Being with you is the only time reality exceeds fantasy."
- "I like the way you smell."
- "We're great for each other."
- "Your company is good for me."
- "I like what you do for me!"

Physical ways:

- a foot massage with lotion anytime
- a body rub with sensory integration activities
- feeding him fruit by hand or by foot
- stroking his entire scalp slowly
- rubbing his hands, twisting his fingers
- sucking his fingers after dinner
- sharing a deep bath by candlelight
- skinny-dipping
- sharing a spaghetti strand
- washing or brushing hair
- shaving legs or face
- sucking fingers/toes
- offering a head massage

Special ways:

- writing original poetry
- making your own card with a personalized note
- watching an adult video together
- sending him a bouquet of flowers
- drawing a picture of how he makes you feel
- playing a special song for him
- dressing up in satin, lace, or leather
- have a scavenger hunt, with you as the prize
- invite him to a romantic picnic with alfresco sex (in the open air)
- leave a note that says, "I wore something special for you today."
- a fake ransom note with cutout letters/pictures pasted on
- couch-spooning while watching a favorite old flick
- become a "sex-knapper" and have a surprise party at a hotel

Be creative. A scavenger hunt, for instance, can be initiated periodically by either party.

Start with a simple handwritten note which you strategically place where you know he'll see it easily. The note might read:

> *"Hi, sweetheart. I just wanted to tell you how much I love you. I'm running out of room here. So go to the cookie jar for your next message."*

Next send him to the refrigerator, the couch, anywhere in the house, invariably ending up in the bedroom. Each note tells him how much you love him and why. Humans never tire of hearing flattery. As long as it's true, you can say the same things over and over again in different ways.

The last note may say, "Look on your bed." Under his pillow, place a small token of your affection. The gift can be as provocative as edible underwear or as practical as a watch, as inexpensive as a Hallmark card or as costly as two tickets to Rio. The point is, you've taken the time to be playful while showing him how much you care. This fanciful attitude spills over into the bedroom.

The Virtue of Seduction

Now that you're in the bedroom, seductively and playfully push your man onto the bed. Offer him a glass of wine that happens to be on the nightstand nearby. Perhaps start with a kiss or by unbuttoning his shirt, slowly, and continue with each delightful piece of clothing until he's bare. He'll follow your lead until neither of you can prolong the anxiety a moment longer. You set a lovable tone for the evening from the moment he found your first note.

Seduction is a wonderful gift. Talking plays a key role for both sexes. The "strong, silent type" from the early silver screen era is not considered sexy by many women anymore. The John Wayne-Clint Eastwood types better listen up! In the nineties, women want a different type. Of course, we don't want the egocentric magpie either, or the one who dotes on us to the point of exaggeration. The real smooth-talking, smooth-acting man, I never quite trust, like the consummate salesman never at a loss for words and whose lines appear practiced and practiced and practiced. Some men can almost talk a woman into a climax with honesty, caring, timing, and personal knowledge.

Honesty is important in seduction. Don't you love it when your man says something sweet and meaningful? It can be as simple as "I can't get enough of you tonight" or "I could just eat you up right now." Even the quiet type is okay as long as he express his feelings periodically. The best times can be before or after lovemaking.

How to Prolong Lovemaking

Most men figure sex is over once they've ejaculated. Even the total gentleman, who makes sure you climax first and then takes his turn, can learn a thing or two about a woman's real needs. If you want to climax more, ask for oral or manual stimulation, and be sure to tell him how much pleasure he "gives" you. Another method is to remain on top after his ejaculation and continue to enjoy more orgasms by rubbing against the warmth and closeness of his body. Even if he's relatively soft, you can learn to climax with the friction of his penis on your clitoris. If he's willing to kiss and stimulate your breasts, this is twice as easy.

The better you are at making requests, without demanding or belittling, the better the sexual encounter will become. Be subtle. The key is to make him feel special during your sexual adventures. Saying things like "You feel wonderful" or "I feel close to you" can add many delicious minutes to your usual routine. By giving honest praise, you can prolong the afterplay. Maybe all you want is to cuddle for a few minutes or to be stroked a little. Once you reassure him that he's the best thing you've ever had he'll be more likely to respond to these requests positively.

Try not to rate his performance during afterplay. Honest exclamations of how you feel are acceptable: "I feel terrific right now" or "You're wonderful!" Remember, this is not the time to offer recommendations for improvement or ask for help with painting the house either. Make suggestions during a nonintimidating time, while watching a hot scene on television or reading a magazine article on the subject. "Let's try that, honey" or "You won't believe what I just read . . . Whaddaya think?" is much less offensive than "You never give me exactly what I want." Besides, it's more effective.

Here's another tactic. Start by reading his *Playboy* issue. He may have already fantasized about trying a few things with you. If you seem interested in experimenting, he'll be more willing to try something new. If he doesn't read *Playboy,* you can always leave this book or a woman's magazine suggestively next to your bed. Leave it open to a particular article. The title alone may entice him to read it. Oh, and don't rule out placing the magazine on the back of the toilet. For some inexplicable reason, men think of bathrooms as their own private library. And if your man wants to try something he finds, be as receptive to the idea as you hoped he would be! What's fair is fair!

The Divine Afterglow

Usually, but not always, women like to bask in the aftermath of good sex. They want to cuddle, talk, sit together, relax, eat, or just hold hands (naked). Men, on the other hand, may want to smoke, get up, or worst of all, roll over and go to sleep. (Now, as I mentioned before, a man secretes chemicals after ejaculation which cause him to be sleepy, so don't be too harsh. However, a few minutes of tenderness won't kill him!) Many men are deficient in this area and almost ruin a perfectly good experience by falling asleep without so much as a "good-night."

If your man could use improvement in this

area, be sweet yet firm. Never demanding. Tell him how important it is that he say a few words. Agree to spend a minimum of five minutes holding and hugging each other. Then add minutes to this whenever possible. A few sincere words is all most females want. Let the stream of consciousness flow after sex during which you confide secrets, recall happy memories, tell jokes, whatever. If accolades and praise are in order, by all means share it. Men should reciprocate. We all need reassurance of our sublime humanness rather than feeling like a vehicle for sexual release. A few minutes of acceptance, warmth, and closeness make all the difference between feeling used and feeling loved.

Bedroom Philosophy

Make sure that your bed is used for two reasons: 1) sleeping or 2) pleasure. Now, pleasure can be reading a book, relaxing, meditating, or sex. Do NOT use the bed as a place to discuss business, problems with the children, or requests for favors. What happens over time is that this anchors in negative feelings that are triggered by just getting into your bed. And that's the last place you want to bring up unpleasant memories.

There's a fine line between intimate talking and talking in general. Of course, couples frequently use the bed to discuss the day's events, what they did, who they saw, how they behaved, and so forth. That's okay. But if your conversations turn into consistent arguments or problem-solving sessions, then I suggest you go to the living room or kitchen to continue your conversation. It doesn't take long before a negative association begins to take hold and affect one's personal attitude in any environment.

Let's say your romantic evenings typically ended on a sour note. Wouldn't you be less likely to initiate them? Pretty soon you might grow resentful. How long would it take before you started to avoid them altogether? This is what happens to couples in long-term relationships who then wonder where the passion went. By anchoring negative feelings instead of the positive ones to the bedroom, couples let it slip by slowly, but surely. The negativity builds on itself until it stifles one's outlook and chips away at the respect, support, and affection couples once had for each other.

Think about it. If the bedroom is the main place you dwell on negative issues, problems with the kids, or business, it's bound to have an effect on your overall outlook each time

144

you step into the room. So make your bedroom the most pleasant, upbeat, warm, caring place it can be—as much as humanly possible. If you haven't started this yet, start **today**!

If you're in a negative pattern, the easiest way to break it is to change the looks of your bedroom physically. Move the furniture around, buy a sexy-looking bedspread or sheets, or add some houseplants or small trees to give it a jungle look. Sit down and talk to your mate about the new philosophy of the bedroom.

Then, for the next forty days, share a positive thought or a good feeling, and vocalize your intent as if it's a reality now. For example, say, "We're the sexiest couple in the whole world." A friend of mine tells her husband, "We're so lucky to have each other!...Let's celebrate the new bedroom look with a back rub...Turn over, you first!" Wouldn't you know? It leads to *spirited sex*!

Is Your Mate Visual, Auditory, Kinesthetic?

Whether or not you've heard of neuro-linguistic programming (NLP), you instinctively know many concepts that make it unique. What is NLP? In short, it's a science that studies the effect of language, verbal and nonverbal, on the nervous system and how behavior is impacted. When you get directions to someone's house, for instance, do you require a map? If so, you're visual. Can you easily understand people's instructions over the telephone? Then you're like me, auditory. Or is it easier if someone drives you there the first time? If so, you're probably kinesthetic.

NLP is a tool to help gain rapport; like many other tools, however, the individual decides how to use it. A fireplace poker, for instance, is supposed to be used to stoke the flames, but it can be used to bop someone on the head. The choice is an individual one. To continue the analogy, let's equate fire to passion. Like my mother always told me, in the beginning of a relationship, there are numerous tall flames. After many years of a solid relationship, mature love is like the fire that has burned down to the coals. Yet, as we all know, coals are hotter than yellow or blue flames. It's those deep, rich, hot coals that make inspired sex. That's what makes the magic. So if NLP can help stoke the sexual coals, I'm gonna use it.

As you gain better rapport with your partner, he will be more likely to make love in new and innovative ways. Exactly how do you go about this? Thankfully, it's very simple. You match various traits and characteristics of your lover. One of the easiest ways to start is by matching his body language. Does he sit with crossed arms and legs? Is he relaxed or tense? How does he tilt his head during intimate conversation? I know this sounds farfetched, but try this: The next time your lover is watching sports on TV, nonchalantly sit in a similar position. You don't need to be so near as to touch him, just where he can perceive your presence. Now, don't be too obvious, but imitate at least two things. Sit there for ten minutes and, if possible, roughly mirror his body position and his breathing pace. Then think sexy thoughts.

The first time I tried this, I was amazed. Within twelve minutes, my partner turned to me and said, "Wanna go upstairs?" (That's one of our signals for wanting sex.) The astounding part is that the basketball game wasn't over yet, and one of his favorite teams was playing. Of course, nothing works all of the time, but why not improve the odds?

Briefly put, you can match or mirror anything from this list, and I guarantee your mate will feel closer to you—even if it's on a subconscious level:

- Tonality (tone of voice, resonance, pitch, volume)
- Distance (space needs)
- Eye Contact (approximate the amount or lack of)
- Facial Expression (smiling, somber, thoughtful, etc.)
- Pace of Speech (quick, slow, combination)
- Body Posture (relaxed, tense, folded, straight)
- Breathing (get in sync by matching exactly)
- Body Changes (calm, fidgety, gross, fine)
- Eye Blinks (slow, fast)
- Language (visual, auditory, kinesthetic)

Last, but not least, is to communicate using the basic visual, auditory, or kinesthetic language mode with your partner. For example, how does your lover typically say good-bye to others? Does he say, "I'll see you later?" "Talk to you soon?" or "Keep in touch?" These VAK words give a deeper insight into an individual's psyche than one might think. They help us *see* our mate in a new *light,* so we can *hear* what he's *telling* us; in this way, we get a *grip* on his *feelings.*

Visual: see, look, clearly, point of view, examine this, focus, picture, colorful, perspective, bright light.

Auditory: hear, listen, sounds like, tell me about it, ear, rings true, clear as a bell, talk, tune in, discuss, off key.

Kinesthetic: feels like, take care, grip, handle the situation, sense, touch, fits for me, hands-on, aware of, pressing.

While all of us use different modes depending on the task at hand, we have a primary representational mode that we use to filter human experiences. According to *Instant Rapport,* 60 percent of the population is visual; just over 20 percent is auditory; slightly under 20 percent is kinesthetic. (By the way, I highly recommend Michael Brook's refreshing and easy-to-read book for anyone interested in learning more about NLP and other communication technologies.) To sum up, the quality of our communication in and out of the bedroom enhances the quality of our lovemaking. If NLP can help keep relationships closer, then I'm all for it!

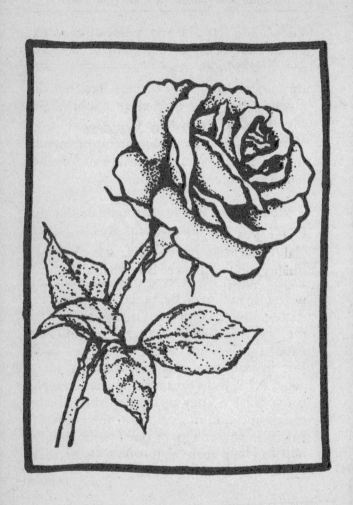

9

Seven Steps to Success

So far I've talked about many aspects of sexuality, including love, lust, self-pleasure, sensuality, and romance. But what about the nitty-gritty of penetration multiple orgasms? Trust me, without the preliminary information, this chapter would have been out of context. After analyzing personal experiences, I've compiled a list of seven steps to successful climaxing:

Step 1) Compatible chemistry

Step 2) Psychological comfort level

Step 3) Plentiful, fabulous foreplay

Step 4) Life-giving breaths

Step 5) Making noises

Step 6) The power of positioning

Step 7) Opening up and letting go

Sex is universal. Yet it's an individual experience. What works for one person may not necessarily work for another. But I suspect we're more alike than different. These seven steps are meant to affirm what you're already doing well and enhance those areas of your lovemaking that could use refinement.

Use whatever feels comfortable to you. Remember, there's no substitution for love. Sex can simply serve lust, or it can transcend desire and merge two dissimilar souls. Think of these progressive steps as practical suggestions to heighten sexual pleasure for you and your partner. If you're serious about wanting to enrich your sex life, try them all. All I can say is, "It works for me!"

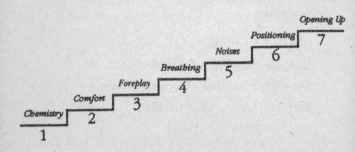

Step One: Compatible Chemistry

First of all, select a man with whom you have a genuine physical attraction. Whether or not you're in love with your partner, it's essential that you feel a chemical harmony when physically close to each other. The feeling of wanting his flesh next to yours is as old as the Garden of Eden. If there's no chemistry, it's like being next to your own brother. When love fades, the same thing happens. It's difficult to create chemistry where none exists, but it's possible to escalate the spark that's already there.

By the way, there are chemicals in your body, called pheromones, that cause the opposite sex to be attracted to you. Once released by your body, this chemical substance influences the physiology and behavior of your mate. Most people don't talk about these little critters lurking around in our bodies, but they're important for the survival of a long-lasting relationship.

If you're attracted to your partner's natural body odor, that's a good sign. In short, make sure your pheromones like his pheromones. By the way, if you've been dating a man for five or six weeks without feeling romantically inclined, then it's probably not meant to be sexual.

Step Two: Psychological Comfort Level

 A woman must first be comfortable with her own body and the ultimate pleasure it can give her. Whether you do this through masturbation or with a partner is incidental. What counts is that you're emotionally complete, relaxed, and whole as a sexual individual. If this remains a stumbling block for you, try one suggestion or exercise at a time, at your own pace, until you are comfortable with your own sexuality.

Discovery & Exploratory Exercises

If masturbation turns you off, there are other alternatives available. One is to ask a partner to stimulate as many places on your body as possible. This is a fun exercise for any couple. The goal is not sexual arousal, although that may occur. In fact, it's more likely to occur if you set a time limit in which you both agree not to have sex, say, for the rest of the afternoon.

One partner becomes the *giver* and agrees to be the silent partner, so to speak, listening and responding as best he or she is able. The *receiver* is only responsible for telling the truth. There is no anxiety about sexual performance during this time because you've already agreed to postpone intercourse.

Instead, the focus is on one person. Think of it as a *Discovery & Exploratory* exercise. Try it for a short period of ten to fifteen minutes in the beginning, building up to longer periods of forty-five to fifty-five minutes maximum. Try this D & E exercise as frequently as you'd like. Twice a month is fine as long as both partners agree and feel it's beneficial.

Let's assume for a moment that you're the receiver. Ask your partner to massage you in various parts of your body, not the breast or genital areas in the beginning. Be sure to use different methods and techniques such as mellow pinching, palm twisting, gentle or rough karatelike chops, kneading, tickling, "typing" or running fingers, and so forth. It's the receiver's job to give feedback such as faster, slower, rougher, more tender. "Easy does it,"

"Oooh, I'd like more of that, please," "Let's move on to a new area," or "I like it better more gentle."

Here are some ideas to use during your D & E exercises. Use them as a springboard for your own imagination. Now jump off and have some fun!

- Start at the top of the head, massaging the scalp, slowly with and without fingertips. Change to a fast and vigorous pace periodically.

- Place a warm washcloth on the back area and move around with the palm of your hand, then in a back-and-forth motion as if you're drying off with a towel.

- Use a cold washcloth and place it in various places on the body for another effect if you're up to it. (With ice chips, it's even chillier!)

- Pour baby powder on the shoulders, inner arms, or buttocks and rub it gently in circles. (Could feel amazingly similar to fur!)

- Take a piece of fleece, silk, or other soft-textured material and move it gently over the stomach, under the armpits, and over the neck until your partner begs for mercy.

- Rub lotion or oil on your mate's feet. Perhaps here, more than anywhere else, you can be rough on the soles and heels. (If unbearably ticklish, it's required.)

- Massage slowly with firm pressure on the bottom of the feet, particularly at the instep and ankle area, which is an erogenous zone for many people. Some massage therapists contend that every nerve in your foot is interconnected with every other part of your body.

- Stroke across the stomach or chest area with a feather, then alternate with sandpaper or some other rough-textured material. Try this on other body parts as well, alternating with warm and cold sensations if desired.

Get the idea? Try a toothbrush, vibrator, body paints, a small pillow, or anything your heart desires so long as your partner gives you permission. A steady mixture of items can integrate more sensations into your lovemaking than you thought possible. Perhaps you've learned about a sensitive area of your partner that you never noticed before. And by all means, trade places. The giver now becomes the receiver.

Not only do *Discovery & Exploratory* exercises

add a new dimension to your sexuality, they also teach partners how to communicate more effectively. In the previous chapter, I talked about positive ways to communicate needs to your mate. This is a nonthreatening environment to practice ways of talking to each other. You may learn this is the best route for both of you to listen to each other as well.

Whether you've been with your mate for a few weeks or a few decades, only you know how comfortable you are with discussing sexual issues. Are you willing to try a new idea you've just read in a magazine or book? It makes sense to go slow in this area. You don't want your sex partner to think he's being used as a guinea pig. Also, you don't want to shock your partner by trying twelve new positions in one night when you've been used to one or two for the past several years. (He might think you've had an affair!) So try one or two new ideas at a time.

How comfortable would you be showing him this manual, for instance? Very comfortable? Somewhat uneasy? Embarrassed? You decide. But first determine if he'll take it as a criticism about his abilities in bed. If you say it tactfully, he'll pay attention: "Honey, you know I enjoy making love with you. Well, tonight I'd like to try something I read that may excite both of us. Would you care to join me?"

Psychological Comfort Profile

Find out where your relationship stands. Take this quick quiz and see how compatible you are. On a scale from 1 to 10, rate the following statements. Consider 1 to be Totally Unlike You and 10 Most Like You (or Your Situation.) Basically, 5 and 6 are neutral numbers and should be avoided unless no other number fits.

___ 1. I talk to my partner/spouse easily about a variety of subjects.

___ 2. When we argue, we come to a resolution in a reasonable amount of time, and then we typically stick with our settlement.

___ 3. I consider my sex partner one of my best friends.

___ 4. We enjoy several mutual interests together. (While we also have separate interests, we devote enough time to our common ones.)

___ 5. When I feel low or blue, my partner usually knows what to do or say. (He either leaves me alone or holds me, etc.)

___ 6. I generally have fun with my partner when we're not in bed.

___ 7. At least once a month, my partner makes me feel "special"—like I really am number one in his life.

___ 8. I can do something silly around my partner and I feel completely at ease about doing so. In other words, he lets me be me.

___ 9. Generally speaking, we have similar tastes in entertainment (i.e., we like the same types of movies and activities).

___ 10. My partner really listens to me when I ask for his undivided attention . . . He tries to understand and accept my viewpoint (although he may not agree with it).

ADD UP TOTAL POINTS: _____

How to Score

If you scored 100 points, get real. Nobody's perfect. You're fooling yourself. Get a life!

If you totaled 70–100 points, you and your mate have **High Compatibility.** He's definitely on the keeper list. You two have more going for you than most couples. You're probably in the top 20 percent. You've got a potential or real soul mate. I bet he makes you feel happy, full, alive, and loved. This is as good as it gets.

If you ended up with 40–69 points, you and your mate have **Fair Compatability.** Add a few things to your "fix list." Your relationship probably works all right most of the time. Still, you feel the struggle to *connect* on a deeper level than "What's for dinner, honey?" Are you bored? You need to recharge either his batteries, your own, or both. Perhaps you deserve better. Start by changing your own behavior—that's the only thing you have total control over anyway.

If you tallied 10–39 points, you have **Low Compatibility.** It's a second-rate relationship at best and needs to go on the "nix list." I suspect you have an arranged, distant association. Even if the sex is good, there aren't very close ties at other times. Are you or your partner afraid of intimacy? Often wonder why you spend much of your life with this man? It's doubtful it'll last unless major changes occur. Do yourself a favor and say good-bye.

Step Three: Plentiful, Fabulous Foreplay

 Foreplay is one of the most essential ingredients for good lovemaking, and too often missing. This step is probably the most difficult one to pin down because it's such an individual thing. What's adequate for you may not be enough for another woman. For that matter, what's enough for you one day may not be adequate the next time.

In my seminars, I hear women needing anywhere from five to forty-five minutes of foreplay. The average seems to be around ten to fifteen minutes. One woman admitted, "Sometimes I never get there." One thing nearly everyone agreed on was this:

Don't watch the news before sex!

Obviously some women take quite a while to get warmed up. Part of it, I believe, goes back to steps one and two. Other reasons may include the following:

- Fatigue
- Hunger

- Pain
- Stress
- Health
- Mood
- Pregnancy
- Past Experiences
- Culture/Upbringing
- Innate Sexual Appetite
- Medication Interference
- Use of Drugs/Alcohol

I think it is important to talk about these briefly and what their impact is on foreplay and sex. When you're tired, hungry, in pain, or stressed out, it influences how you're going to approach a sexual encounter. The same goes for your partner, of course, so be sympathetic. If you're only a little tired, it's okay to make love without wanting an orgasm. Sometimes you feel loving but don't feel up to the whole trip. Just explain it to your partner ahead of time so he won't expect animal passion. You might say, "I'd like to have sex, but I'm a little bushed... I probably won't be my usual lustful love monster... so please don't take it personally when I say, 'Your turn'... That'll be you're cue to come. Okay?"

Obviously you can control some of the barriers rather easily. For example, you can sleep, eat, and take an analgesic, and shortly thereafter be revived, to a greater or lesser degree, and enjoy healthy and happy sex. If your pain or health problem is major, it should be discussed with your personal physician.

If you're angry with your partner, or vice versa, then that's another story. It's important to discover the cause of the interference. Share your feelings with each other after you've meditated on it for a while by yourself. Sometimes we get upset at the moment; but in the cosmic scope of things, it's a petty issue. So work through those by yourself. If you bother your partner with every single concern, your mate won't listen to the big issues. It's like crying "Wolf" too often. When the wolf really comes, nobody's there to support you.

Okay, so you've chosen your issue and you need to work through the anger; otherwise resentment will seep into the bedroom. Other emotions play a role in sex as well. Fear, anxiety, and previous flops are also key barriers in preventing orgasms. Did you know that your testosterone level goes down when you're anxious? Remember, testosterone is responsible for your sex drive. Sometimes just telling your partner some of your fears will reduce the stress enough to climax. He may have a few fears, anxieties, and past failures of his own; your openness may lead to greater intimacy.

Mood is a strange phenomenon. We can control it, whether we realize it or not, by thinking positive or negative thoughts. Sometimes one thought triggers bad memories or feelings prior to a sexual encounter. Once I went ahead and had intercourse in spite of a negative thought that had just popped into my mind. Within six or seven minutes, my lover asked, "What's wrong?" My private thought wasn't something I felt like sharing at the time, so I simply said, "My head's not in the right place right now." So we talked, drank wine, and played Boggle for a while. Within an hour, I was hornier than ever. Thanks to an understanding lover and my ability to admit the truth, we shared wonderful, dreamy lovemaking that day.

About pregnancy. While expecting, I've experienced the entire range—from being exceptionally horny to not interested in sex at all. Each woman is different; so just tell your partner how you're feeling. Tell him it's temporary in either case and that your hormones are going crazy for a while, but they'll be sane again shortly. The outcome of a precious child is worth a short-term interruption or change in your sex life. And if a man can't understand that simple concept, tell him to stick it!

If you take prescription medication, engage in heavy drinking, or consume drugs on a regular basis, then don't be surprised if your sex life is adversely affected. Sure, a few glasses of wine can be relaxing and enhance an encounter. But alcohol, as well as many other drugs, is a depressant and will decrease your ability to feel sensations. Of course, it can also prevent the man from getting an erection at all if he has consumed large amounts. I'm not trying to be preachy, I'm just giving you the facts. Even stimulants that can seemingly give a temporary aphrodisiac effect can ruin a satisfying sex life in the long run.

The most difficult influences upon your ability to enjoy foreplay and sex are preadulthood factors such as growing-up experiences, and how your family discussed the issue or didn't discuss it. These types of experiences impact our feelings and attitudes in a big way. Furthermore, if early rape, incest, or other sexual molestation has occurred, it can be extremely difficult to relax and enjoy a man. It may take years of trusting a man and/or years of therapy to undo the emotional damage caused by heartless humans earlier in life.

The Importance of Kissing

Kissing is a unique, special mode of communication. A definite turn-on. If a man hasn't kissed you on the neck, shoulders, forehead, breasts, butt, toes, armpit, back, earlobe, or behind the knees—you haven't really been kissed adequately. (Minimally, he should choose seven out of ten places.) And let's not forget to return the favor!

There's a connection between how someone kisses and how he'll perform intercourse or cunnilingus. Don't you agree? There are exceptions to every rule, but on the whole, a good kisser makes a wonderful lover. Describe a good kisser. We all probably have personal quirks, but why did so many women love Kevin Costner's line in *Bull Durham* about long, soft, deep, slow kisses? It's universal.

It's possible to teach a man how to kiss the way you prefer, but the problem is that most men are too set in their ways or too egotistical to be told that they need improvement in this area. Also, it's easier if the man gets his training early in life, preferably as a teenager. Teenagers are more willing to experiment than a man in his thirties or forties. (I've been told that once past fifty, they revert to the explorative teenager mentality. Great!)

Kissing is an essential part of foreplay. To a woman, kissing shows that a man cares. More important, it helps rev up her sexual motor. Have you ever noticed that when your lover touches your body without kissing, you lubricate less quickly than if he kisses you without touching your body? This probably depends on one's mood, but no doubt women like to be kissed.

By listing several types of kisses, in no way do I want to imply that this is a complete catalog. It's simply a way to show a relation between kissing and foreplay. Here are six basic types.

1) Short, closed-mouth pecks

2) Soft, open-mouthed without tongue

3) Soft, open-mouthed Frenching

4) Hard, open-mouthed without tongue

5) Hard, open-mouthed Frenching

6) Playful tongue flicking

1) Isn't it important to know what kind of kisses you like? Personally, I like most kisses as long as they're not too wet, too hard, or too artificial. Nobody likes someone who slobbers all over her. Short, closed-mouth kisses are never too wet. To me, they signal that my mate

is interested in showing affection. He may just need a hug or the return of a few pecks, or he may be telling me that he wants to make love. Whenever in doubt, just ask. These kisses can also be used after a passionate encounter. A few pecks on my forehead, neck, arms, or back shows me he loves me for me—not just because I was terrific in bed. Don't you feel a warm glow inside when your partner offers a few pecks beforehand or as part of the afterglow?

2) Next is the soft, open-mouthed kiss without tongue. It is perhaps the sweetest kiss, a sign of affection with more of an emotional punch than a briefer peck. Usually this is used as a definite prelude to sex. Haven't you ever used this style in the heat of passion because you're too ecstatic to concentrate on using your tongue? It's the sensation of a warm, moist mouth next to yours that counts. Mouth-to-mouth closeness is just what the doctor orders at times.

3) Category three is terrific as a lead-up to sex play because it tends to get your juices flowing fairly quickly. Gentle, open-mouthed French kisses are the "meat and potatoes" of kissing as far as I'm concerned. In all frontal face-to-face positions, this kiss adds sensationally to intercourse and can be used throughout

a sexual union, if you desire. It's also great during foreplay. For me, this kiss matches my favorite style of lovemaking, which can be described as a medium-paced, magically mellow, floating style.

4) Hard, open-mouthed kisses without tongue have their place as well. They indicate animalistic ardor, a lustful passion. When mixed with the other styles, these can be very effective. These kisses also tend to speed up the rhythms of pelvic gyrations.

5) With French kissing added to the hard, open-mouthed style, the kisses become symbolic of what is happening in the lower part of one's body. Deep tongue is like a second penetration, imitating or directing what goes on elsewhere. Consequently, the pelvic thrusts become faster, more frantic, more beastly. When his tongue is inserted deeper, so his penis seems to penetrate farther into the vagina.

6) Finally, playful tongue flicking is one of the most precious types of kisses. Our sexuality is as much a part of our lives as getting up in the morning, feeding the dog, or going to work. And I like a little humor mixed in with those activities every now and then. When your mate and you exchange playful kisses, don't you feel happy and lighthearted, ready

to meet the world squarely? If you maintain some playfulness in your kissing, you're more likely to try news things. By doing so, you keep sex from becoming stale and repetitious.

All in all, I suppose there's an infinite number of ways to kiss. Believe it or not, I can usually tell how our lovemaking will proceed by how my mate kisses me during foreplay. His style sets the stage for a round of animal passion or a more mellow, magical night. To sum up, kissing has a direct impact on the progression of foreplay and eventually on the sensations of intercourse. To enjoy sex to its fullest, I recommend a mixture of kisses to match your specific sexual need at a particular moment in time.

The Value of Touching

Foreplay consists of mainly kissing and touching. As any physical therapist knows, massage is good for the body, mind, and soul. Hard pressure relaxes our body while light pressure excites or stimulates us. Stick with deep pressure for long enough to give the desired effect, then change to light, superficial touches. Alternating soft and tender with hard and rough usually has a positive effect. Alternate fast with slow, deep with superficial, strong with tender, for even better results.

Check it out with your partner, though. You can do this either verbally—"Do you like this?"—or by observing bodily reactions such as his eyes closing, pupils dilating, penis becoming erect, or legs stiffening. Some people hate to be touched lightly, claiming that they're too ticklish. Others don't like deeper pressure, saying it hurts. Strike a happy medium, but vary your touches to some degree.

Traditional foreplay primarily consists of back, breasts, butt, and clitoral and vaginal stimulation. Again, tell your partner if he's too rough or if you'd rather he be rougher. Be sure to state it positively: "Do that again—but slower, softer." That statement is much more likely to get the results you want than "You never do it right!" He'll take that as a criticism. Who wouldn't? Respond to his suggestions as well. You can ask him to state them in a positive "do it again" manner.

About breasts: Interestingly enough, no two people are alike. Even identical twins have pet techniques that work for one but not the other. Medium pressure with a firm open hand is what some women prefer during the warm-up stage. It's true that a woman's nipple has a direct hot line to her clitoris. The closer I am to orgasm, the rougher my lover can be with my nipples. If a man twists your nipple between his thumb and forefinger during the heat of passion, you may love it, unaware of exactly what he's doing. But if he tried the same technique too early, it could be painful. Just say, "Not yet." A clearer message might be "Wait until I'm closer to orgasm."

In spite of the fact that breasts are an effective trigger for turning women on, many men are clutzy at touching them—squeezing, biting, grabbing, poking, or gnawing too hard. We must teach them that a variety of slow up-and-down or circular motions, kneading with increased firmness, seems to work best. Again, this is such an individual preference—so talk it over with your partner.

Tender sucking on nipples is also great for arousal. After a few minutes, tempestuous nibbling and kissing may be acceptable. What a wonderful way to begin foreplay. Sometimes this works for both sexes. Some men love to have their nipples suckled; others find it distasteful. Like women, each person has his own preference. Explore and discover!

Food and Foreplay

Food, drink, and sex go together like snow-skiing and Jacuzzi dips, as long as it's in the proper proportion. If you have too much food on hand, your sexual encounter could turn into a food frenzy. It's nice to have a cool drink on the nightstand. Don't you get thirsty half-way through a long, passionate episode? Make sure the glass is close enough to grab easily during a rest period. It's nice for the partner on top to take a sip, then kiss the one on bottom, letting a little liquid into your lover's mouth. (Not too much or he'll choke!)

Food can be used creatively. Grapes work well in the mouth or the vagina, as do other pieces of fruit. Of course, whipping cream has been touted as the perfect sex food! All I know is that it depends on you and your mate's preference. Never insert something dangerous into your vagina. My gynecologist objects to Alka-Seltzer in the vagina, for example. Always ask your doctor if you're concerned about the potential effects of something you're doing. Don't be embarrassed about asking questions. We deserve to get our money's worth. Remember, no question is a stupid question. Wouldn't it be worse to get an infection?

Offbeat Foreplay Ideas

Toe sucking may not sound appealing at first, but try it at least once. After a bath, shower, or fun in a hot tub, it's the perfect time to suggest that your mate use your toes as Popsicles. It's a real turn-on for most women who have tried it. To have a man massage your toes in his mouth is a marvelous adventure. Don't knock it till you've tried it.

Another foreplay idea revolves around the buttocks. Equally a turn-on for both sexes, the butt is a great place to warm up your partner. It's a terrific visual source of arousal as well. Before or during intercourse, don't you like it when your partner grabs your butt firmly, one cheek in each hand? Some people like harder pressure or slapping mildly or even stronger kneading. This manual does not discuss S/M (sadomasochism) or B & D (bondage and discipline).

For a variation on a theme, try this. In the middle of a romantic interlude, when the man is lying facedown, start by crawling on top of his back, rubbing it with the front of your body and hands. Moving downward, end up with your breasts in the crack of his butt and your genitals somewhere midleg. Your clitoris can be stimulated by the friction of your movements while your breasts reap the benefit as you play with his butt. Somehow the feeling of your chest on his butt is a turn-on for both people. Experiment in this position for a while to see if you like it. Trust me, it's worth a try.

The point is, foreplay is an individual thing. Two consenting adults should explore a variety of ideas. The purpose of foreplay is to arouse both people for successful and comfortable penetration and/or oral sex. Gratification from oral sex may be considered foreplay or the pinnacle of the sexual encounter. It all depends on one's point of view. In short, adequate foreplay is something to be discovered and rediscovered with your partner throughout your relationship.

Lace, Silk, or Leather?

Does your man like to see you in lace? Does he get hot when you wear tight leather pants? Or is he the silky, soft type? As I mentioned before, a male's sexual arousal is triggered by visual things. Why not take advantage of it? The woman who enjoys dressing up for herself and her man can go to a lingerie store (like Frederick's of Hollywood or Victoria's Secret) for a variety of styles. If you're interested, try a "merry widow," lacy camisole with matching panties, a negligee, long gown, or garter belt with stockings. If you like how you feel, imagine the pleasure you'll give your partner!

If you're not used to this, start with a more

traditional nightgown. Then get comfortable in your new outfit. Wear it for a few hours, vacuum a room or do light housework, get natural until it becomes a part of you. When your mate first sees you in it, act nonchalant. Pretend to be reading a magazine, then ask, "How was your baseball game, dear?" You just might have dessert before dinner.

One word of caution. Don't expect a prologue to sex every time you wear something sexy. If your mate says he's tired or needs to unwind first, let him. Continue to wear the outfit. Simply put on one of your mate's shirts over it and continue with your normal routine. Every so often, tease him by flipping up the bottom of his shirt to let him see what you're wearing. Sooner or later, he'll be rested and ready. You can make dressing up part of your foreplay repertoire. Eventually your lover will ask, "When are you gonna wear that lacy red negligee again?"

Fabulous Foreplay

I've heard many wide-ranging responses to the question "What kind of foreplay do you like best?" "Just lying next to him, drawing in his scent." "Breasts. He has to touch my breasts ... It's that simple." "Talking to get on the same wavelength." We all have our own preferences.

Have you ever asked your partner what foreplay he likes best? Remember, assumptions may lead to trouble. Why not be up-front and clear? Here's another suggestion. If you can afford it, visit a massage therapist who works with couples and is willing to teach you stimulating techniques. Some charge the normal hourly rate for this long-lasting treasure. If this is unaffordable, go to the library and get a book on the subject of massage.

Remember that good foreplay, like spirited sex, is also 90 percent mental. When the mood is right, a couple can enjoy long intervals of foreplay. If you're comfortable with your current pattern, great. If not, it's easy to break the mold. Offer something fun and pleasurable. Like Mikey and his cereal, your partner will like it!

Step Four: Life-giving Breaths

 Because of modern-day stress, most women in our culture have long forgotten how to breathe properly. Unknowingly, many of us have actually reversed the natural air flow direction, thereby increasing stress in our body. As I've said before, anxiety interferes with our testosterone level and can decrease our sex drive.

Long, deep breaths are a simple healing breath we did as a child, the type animals and primitive societies still do today. Reeducate yourself to do this simple deep breathing, and the benefits will amaze you in and out of the bedroom!

How to Begin Transforming Breaths

As you inhale, push your abdomen outward. Your muscles push the diaphragm down and create a vacuum in the lung cavity. As you exhale, pull the abdomen inward. Your diaphragm moves up and creates a pressure on your lung cavity, causing air to be fully expelled. Each inhale and exhale should be as long as possible. Gradually increase the total length to eight to sixteen counts. An important note: Close your eyes while you do this to get the greatest benefits.

If you can do this for a minimum of three minutes within an hour before sex, it will give you a calm demeanor and focused energy. Be sure to breathe fully during crescendos of lovemaking. Of course, the ultimate goal is to breathe properly throughout your entire day, thus relieving the normal buildup of stress.

The Benefits of Breathing

It would be hard to overemphasize the importance of breathing properly during sex, or any other time for that matter. Oxygen in our lungs not only keeps us alive, but also stimulates our senses. The temperature for greatest mental alertness is reportedly around sixty-eight degrees. Think about keeping your bedroom at this ideal temperature. We commonly inhale more deeply in cool weather.

Breathing fully enhances sexual pleasure. Any athlete knows that proper breathing increases physical performance, and yoga experts maintain one can reach physical and spiritual "highs" through proper breathing techniques. I'd add sexual highs as well.

If you find yourself holding your breath periodically during sex, it's a sign of tension. Likewise, shallow breathing may mean you're trying too hard or you're not totally relaxed. By the way, if your mouth is slightly open, your wrists and knees bent, then you will automatically be more relaxed.

Once practiced, life-giving breaths become a habit, allowing for full appreciation of stimulated senses. It is especially important to breathe sufficiently during deep thrusts and orgasms. Personally, I love to hear the sounds of my own breathing. It's like a symphony to my partner. He genuinely enjoys hearing my buildup to the plateau phase and orgasmic release throughout an encounter. Think about it. A rapid breathing pace signals crescendos so your partner can better match your impulses. Then there's a natural, mellow slowdown of pace between orgasms. Ample steady breaths increase your physical sensation. Happily, it's easy to learn.

Step Five: Making Noises

Like breathing, making noises is an important step in the realization of multiple or sequential orgasms. Sex sounds are natural. Perhaps they're primitive, but they shouldn't be considered un- ladylike or unsophisticated. On the contrary, love noises can become as pleasant as Beethoven's Ninth to your lover's ears. As you let out noises, you exchange energy with your partner, letting him know the depth or tempo of rhythms with each new release. Each sound strikes an inner cord and relates how you're feeling. Noises let your partner know when he delights you!

You may have your own personal repertoire of moans, groans, cries, and phrases. Usually short phrases do the trick:

"That's good!"

"Oh, God, oh, oh!"

"Aaaaaaaaaaaaaaaah!"

"Perfect!"

"Ummmmmmmm!"

"I love this!"

"Ooooooooooooooh!"

"Oh, sweetheart!"

Well, I think you get the picture. Can simple moans and groans really increase your pleasure? You bet your voice box! One time, I blurted out "Damn you" during a particularly passionate lovemaking encounter. Our sex had been ultraterrific, so my lover knew it was a compliment. But afterward he asked, "Why did you cuss at me?" "You were too wonderful!" I said honestly. "There's no such thing!" was his comeback. Now all I have to do to get him aroused is repeat those two words, "Damn you," with a particular intonation. (Remember *anchoring* from the last chapter?) The point is, as long as we say something affectionately and sincerely, it will usually come across in that light.

Nothing quite reaches the inner core of a man's heart as much as hearing his name during the heat of passion. A simple "Oh, Tom" can works wonders for his arousal. Just remember the risks involved. If you accidentally say, "Oh, Bill," you can kiss his erection goodbye. Be absolutely sure of yourself.

Also, how comfortable are you making any kind of noises in front of your mate? My advice is to incorporate a few sounds into your sex life because it enhances your own experience. Start softly with a few moans (sincere ones) if it's not a part of your usual style. Then slowly add volume and variety until it becomes more natural to make noises. To be totally honest, talk with him first. Tell him that you'd like to start making more noise during sex, that you feel a little silly about it, but you'd like to try it out. He may surprise you with his response.

Simple moans and groans do several things to increase your pleasure. First, it lets him know that he's pleasing you. And secondly, the expression of bliss keeps you in the present. When people disassociate themselves from the encounter, then sex becomes mechanical. Many people purposely go "out of body" to avoid experiencing what is happening or to avoid the vulnerable feelings that can accompany great sex. To be present, be sure to moan, cry, grunt, or whine as the mood strikes. Stay in tune with how each physical perception is affecting and pleasing you. Discover a distinct sound for each new sensation.

Step Six: The Power of Positioning

 For good results, try a number of positions during lovemaking. This does not necessarily mean you need to try hundreds of ways as described in the Kama Sutra. Rather, experiment with various tilts and angles of penetration to discover the many that give you pleasure. The basic four is still the place to start. Then vary leg positions: open, closed, bent, straight. If your lover doesn't move his piston to suit you, you can always move your cylinder. Don't worry, he'll follow.

If you're interested, there are plenty of books on the market that specialize in showing a variety of positions. Many of them are hardly worth the trip except to satisfy your curiosity or prove your physical agility.

In rock and roll, there are only a few core rhythms and patterns; the rest are variations on a theme. Likewise, there are only a few basic sexual positions:

1) Frontal (face-to-face)
2) Sideways (legs in between)
3) Rear entry (man from behind)
4) Astride (sitting)

1) Let's discuss some of the advantages and disadvantages of these positions. Frontal positions include all face-to-face postures where one partner has both thighs between the other's. The traditional missionary position was so named by the natives of Polynesia, who usually made love in a squatting position. They considered Western missionaries' man-on-top position amusing and strange. They called it the "missionary" position almost as a term of derision. If it is the only position a man likes to use, then it deserves its bum rap. But mixing it up with other styles is fine, and there are a couple of valid reasons for using it on a periodic basis.

If the man is on top, and if he positions himself slightly forward, the base of his penis stimulates his partner's clitoral area above the vagina, thus making orgasm easier. With the woman on top, she can easily control rhythm, depth of penetration, thrust power, and so forth. It is comfortable for her, and the man can caress her breasts and buttocks at will. The comfort factor is especially important if the man weighs a great deal more than the woman. This position relieves the man of the performance responsibility, that is, it can be a psychological relief for males not to control the entire scenario from start to finish. Last, but not least, there is better stimulation potential of the clitoris in this position.

Also, in this configuration, it is easier for the woman to position herself to maximize pleasure against a man's pubic bone, creating a sexually exciting tension with each movement. Some men are able to shift from "tough" to "tender" more easily when the woman is on top because the reactions and feel of her are more readable.

2) In the *Joy of Sex*, Alex Comfort refers to this sideways position as "flanquette" where she lies facing him with one of her legs between his. This can stimulate the woman's clitoris if the man applies pressure with his thigh. Many people find this position useful to switch from the other more popular positions.

3) If the man penetrates the woman from

behind, he can manually stimulate her clitoris effortlessly. Alex Comfort has it listed under its French name, "croupade." For the highly spirited, this position—sometimes called "doggie style"—provides a vigorous, animalistic approach to sex. While all right for a change of pace, there is a loss of intimacy without the face-to-face encounter. It is not possible to kiss or look into each other's eyes. Half-rear entries are called "cuissade," where her back is turned to him and one of her legs is between his, facing away.

4) "Astride" refers to a sitting or kneeling type of position, with the legs typically around the other's hips. It can be a frontal or rear-entry position, but different enough to mention it separately. The greatest benefit is that this position offers deeper penetration than any other. A woman can rub her chest or head against the man's face more gracefully. A perfect match-up of body size becomes less of an issue here. For some women, this position has given them the best sex they've ever known!

A brief word needs to be said about positions as they relate to oral sex. The popular "sixty-nine" (*soixante-neuf* in French) refers to the head-to-toe position while both parties are performing oral sex. Mutual "mouth music" is usually enjoyable; but if either party is going to climax, it is advisable to take turns. The man, in particular, may be inadvertently bitten if a woman becomes too excited during orgasm.

While I can have orgasms in a variety of positions, I do have my favorites, especially to experience multiple and sequential orgasms. My two basic positions for this are: 1) With me on top, usually starting out with my knees bent, like a frog. You might say this is not a pretty picture, but the euphoric feelings override any sense of pride. 2) Facing my lover, astride, as he sits with his back against the couch or something sturdy. My legs can either be wrapped around him or dangle to the side, knees bent. Something else may work for you, but I wanted to share what suits me best. We know that the pubococcygeal muscle is on the frontal side of the vagina; it may get the greatest friction in the positions described above.

One last thing about the power of positioning: You have the right to suggest a change anytime. If it suits you, invent pet names for particular positions. If you're fond of gymnastics, for example, you could say, "Let's do the reverse gainer" whenever you wanted to make love head to toe. Try it, you may like it! Have fun with naming your favorite positions!

Step Seven: Opening up and Letting Go

To open yourself up, you have to learn to truly receive what your partner has to give. This is an art in itself. Being receptive is not the same as taking. It's not spacing out into passivity. A passive partner is a boring partner. Your partner should allow you to give whatever you choose to give. Each partner needs to have the opportunity to receive. If partners give continuously, they eventually feel cheated. True receiving, though, is without greed. Instead, it means paying attention to your partner to make the experience a mutual one. Simply put, be enthusiastic whether you take the lead or not.

Likewise, giving is not the same as controlling someone. To give freely never violates the comfort level of another individual. Giving openly is being sensitive to the needs and desires of the receiver. The giver can then adjust to the other's mood. This pure giving has no air of desperation or compulsion. Many insecure people feel compelled to give continuously so they can feel needed, loved, or valuable. Ideally, partners take turns taking the initiative. Better yet, giving and receiving become so intermeshed, it's difficult to distinguish between the giver and the receiver. When there is no clear-cut giver and receiver, you've truly succeeded!

Opening up mainly refers to a psychological phenomenon. However, I need to add a few important physical steps as well. At the risk of sounding mundane, a woman needs to make sure she empties her bladder before she has sexual intercourse. Sometimes you may even need to empty it again in the middle of sex, especially if you've had tea or coffee beforehand. When you come back, be sure to stroke him tenderly a few times or go to a favorite foreplay move. Trust me, it's important to be free of worry if you want to have multiple or sequential orgasms. You have to open yourself up totally. In the back of your mind, if you think your bladder isn't empty, what do you suppose happens? You tense up just a little. Don't let a few seconds of embarrassment stop you from asking, "Can we take a quick break?" If you don't, you're undermining your own potential for pleasure.

Putting It All Together

Intercourse should not be painful. If it is, perhaps you're not lubricated properly. If pain is regular, consult your physician. However, most women experience some discomfort every now and then during intercourse. Sometimes this is because his penis penetrated too deeply, too quickly for your vagina to stretch accordingly. You might say, "Go slow" or "I'm not ready yet; can we kiss/pet more first?" As mentioned before, your vagina can accommodate any size penis. Sometimes the angle of penetration hits close to your urethra, creating a sharp, quick pang. (This can happen if your bladder is full.)

I want to talk about another pleasure/pain phenomenon. Have you ever wondered if it's true that pleasure and pain are close to the same thing? Evidently both feelings are centered in the same part of the brain. You'll know exactly what I'm talking about once you experience this internal tender spot.

I'm not sure if this is the famous "G-spot," named after gynecologist Ernst Graffenburg, or not. Truth is, no one is sure about its existence since it remains scientifically unproven. Sometimes called the Graffenburg spot, it has been described as a lump on the frontal wall of the vagina about one to two inches inside the opening. The theory says that the spot is the equivalent of a male prostate gland. Although there are no conclusions on its validity, direct stimulation to the G-spot is supposed to lead to greater sexual enjoyment.

All I know is, there's a spot that makes me absolutely crazy with pleasure when my partner touches it repeatedly. It's a particularly sensitive place that I describe as my innermost core. At first, it's slightly uncomfortable. For one-millionth of a second, I swear I can't take it another moment. Then, all of a sudden, magic!

The point is, if you feel only slight discomfort, you may want to continue. Slowly, at first, until you get used to the sensation and what ultimate pleasure it will bring you. Of course, if you feel great discomfort, change positions or make your partner aware by verbally stating what the trouble is (in a positive way such as "Can we go slower please?"). Anyway, when there's deep penetration at a particular angle, I feel extra hot. Each thrust purposely hits my pleasure/tender spot. At first, there's an almost imperceivable discomfort. When I continue for several more seconds, I go "beyond" the tenderness and I'm in orgasmic paradise! I call it my *Heavenly Orgasm*, because that's what it feels like.

If I'm relaxed, breathing properly, and making noises, I can continue in this celestial state for quite a while. In fact, once he hits my "spot," he doesn't want to get off of it—unless I make a conscious decision that I've had enough. Not that I strive for a certain type of orgasm, but if I've had several orgasms, I usually add a truly explosive one, the kind that sends shock waves through my entire body, leaving me paralyzed with tingling sensations.

If I purposely strive for any type of orgasm, it eludes me. That's the real trick to all of this. Never aim for a particular sensation; just enjoy.

Brainstorming Ways to Open up and Let Go

Whether you lean toward the visual, auditory, or kinesthetic when you make love, here are some suggestions for letting go during sex:

VISUALIZATION

- Look at your mate's facial features
- Think about specific pictures in your mind, like a beach scene
- Envision what an outsider would say the sex act looked like
- Visualize a melting image of two inter-meshing bodies

- Think of a *Playgirl* centerfold (Burt Reynolds or whoever)
- Look at the mirror on the ceiling
- See how the light reflects on your partner
- Notice body shapes or spaces and how they fit together

SCRIPTING (SELF-TALK)

- Continually talk to yourself to keep you in the present
- Tell yourself how much pleasure you give your partner
- Think of dirty words, harsh language, or commands if it suits you
- Use comic relief: "You Tarzan, me Jane!"
- Silently say, "I love you," "I want you," etc.
- Pretend your mate is a symbolic *Everyman* and talk to him

TOUCHING/BONDING

- Think only about what he feels like next to you

- Concentrate on distinct sensations in a specific locale
- Soak up the global sensations of the encounter
- Grab his hair or scalp, gently, and pull
- Offer a friendship squeeze of hands
- Practice your Kegel exercises on your partner
- Tickle his arms or back or whatever

In summary, to have sequential, motionless, or multiple orgasms, we must let go of prescriptive methods and ritualistic techniques. Instead, attend to the energy at hand, opening up to the reality of the encounter. This means resting and slowing your pace intermittently. Touch or talk tenderly at these times, and be aware of the emotional energy flowing between you. Your success is more dependent upon you being geared to the present energy level than to preprogrammed techniques. If you have a fixed idea of ever-increasing arousal, you have to let go of it. Anything designed to guarantee an orgasm will surely fall short. If you strive for an "ideal" of perfect sex, it will elude you.

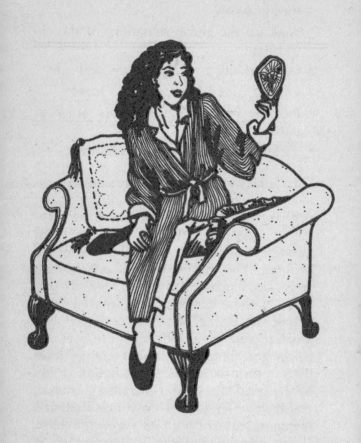

10

Start the Sparks!

You've definitely come a long way, baby—
from your mother's womb to your lover's la-
goon—and you're now ready for heightened
sexual pleasure. Bravo! On your road to becoming the finest individual you can be, I'm
glad you've incorporated sexuality as part of
the game plan. Without sex, we wouldn't be
here. With animated and loving sex, we become humanized in a very primitive, yet profound, way. It's a marvelous, metaphysical
experience.

If you've been paying attention, then you
know what beliefs you need to assimilate into
your private system of convictions. You can do
it. First, take charge of your own orgasm. Secondly, accept the belief that inspired sex is 90

percent mental; and, lastly, embrace your physical self. Trust me, you'll be creating *female fireworks* sooner than you think!

Food and Fun

Making love is a diversified as eating. Sometimes, don't you just feel like a snack? Another day, only a seven-course meal hits the spot. Whether it's an appetizer, a side dish, an entrée, or dessert, enjoy whatever you're eating. Think of sex in the same way.

The trick is to sit down to the table with your mate and order a similar meal. If you always want to go to fancy restaurants while your mate prefers McDonald's, there's bound to be conflict. In this case, both parties can compromise. Your exquisite tastes could learn to appreciate old-fashioned meat and potatoes. On the other hand, your partner could dress up and take you to the Ritz every now and then, right?

So it is with sex. If you always demand a full-course meal, it could negatively affect you partner's sexual desires. He may not initiate because of performance anxiety. Never criticize your mate for wanting a quick snack occasionally. Sooner or later, he'll stop wanting the entire meal. And don't think it's only men who just want snacks. Some women are hooked on it. They've gotten into the snacking habit and call it a meal. Schedule your time for that seven-course meal at least every month. Life's too short to miss out on this libidinous enchantment.

Both sexes may periodically forget the simple joys of spending half the day in bed—stroking, holding, loving, kissing, or petting. Parents, in particular, need to make an extra effort to get away by themselves, even for a day, and focus on each other. You manage to get a sitter for those special occasions, so why not get one for the worthwhile purpose of maintaining a good relationship? It's worth the effort and the money. Try this once every three months for starters. Believe me, you'll see the difference it makes in your lovemaking!

Remember, sex is like food. Some nights you feel like a hamburger. Some nights you want lobster. It goes the same for your mate. Communicate what you want, and then be willing to compromise. There's an old joke about a man who brags that sex is great with his wife, even comparing their lovemaking to filet mignon. Then he adds, "But who wants to eat steak every night?" Bad joke.

Personally, I believe you can enjoy different kinds of meals with the same person. Enjoy steak, sword-fish, chicken, hamburger, frog's legs, pheasant, roast duck—something different every night for a month. It all depends on one's imagination, mood, and love for the other person. In short, there's no aphrodisiac like love!

A Menu for Loving

Appetizers:	Side Dishes:
foot massage	*hand lotion*
toe sucking	*edible gel*
love nibbles	*vibrator*
body caresses	*French tickler*
back rubbing	*tantalizing lingerie*
butt bites	*dressing up*
head massage	*role-playing*
arm tickling	*edible underwear*
butt massage	*seductive body paints*
butterfly kisses (eyelash flutters)	*silk, lace, leather*
	playful sensory toys
soft, slow kisses	*washcloths/ feathers*

Appetizers:
body tickles

animalistic kisses
behind-the-knee
bites

Side Dishes:
homemade sex
gadgets
nearby ice chips
warm/cold water

Entrées:
mutual
masturbation
face-to-face
intercourse
doggie-style
penetration
sideways/sliding
style
straddle
intercourse
cozy cunnilingus
delectable fellatio
sensual sixty-nine
erotic fantasies

Desserts:
alluring whipped
cream
lascivious
mangoes
seductive
strawberries
grapes in the
vagina
sweet, luscious
hugs
cuddly squeezes
chilled champagne
"hot lip" espresso
homemade milk
shakes

Smile, and the World Smiles with You

Good luck on your new adventure! Before
you start on it, be dead sure you want to take

it. "Of course I want to!" you say. Unless you're enthusiastic and confident, you wouldn't even want to go on a picnic, let alone start on a journey destined to change the course of your sex life for the rest of your existence!

When your appetite gains a competitive edge, you enjoy meals more. This adventure means living to the fullest, exposing your deepest emotional and physical appetites to your partner. It's a little scary at first. But once you experience *spirited sex,* you'll never want to turn back. At least you'll never be completely satisfied if you do.

Remember, a playful attitude of fun and discovery increases the possibility of success and heightens sexual enjoyment. Try one thing at a time. Don't rush into anything you're not comfortable with. As the saying goes: *"Inch by inch, it's a cinch. Yard by yard, it's hard!"* I have every confidence that you'll succeed on your journey to sexual bliss!

Dare to Be Adventurous!

Dare to be an adventurer and you'll taste the delights of orgasmic paradise! Dare to try the advice in this book! Keep a positive outlook on life in general. Remember, your sex life is an extension of your personality! Active, spirited lovemaking can be reached more easily if you maintain an upbeat outlook about every aspect of your life. If you aspire to greater sexual adventures, they will meet you halfway. The trick is to find the pathway for the other half. This book is your tool, your personal guide, to that pathway.

Awaken the sleeping adventurer within you! Finding a new sexual awareness brings new treasures into the rest of your life as well. You'll find yourself more able to concentrate, to be creative, to work efficiently, and to love more freely. You'll be more comfortable with life, with people, with ideas. Another interesting thing. The more you find to give sexually, the more you're able to receive. Share this adventure with your partner, and watch your delight multiply. Once you're willing to open up and try new things, the thrill of orgasmic ecstasy is yours!

One Last Piece of Advice

While I wish it were otherwise, there's no mythical maiden who comes down to teach women the best way to have sex. We have to figure it out for ourselves. But, hopefully, you can use this book as a motivator to enhance your sexual relationship. In the first chapter, I asked you to reconsider how fulfilling your current sex life is, and challenged you to discover ways to enhance it. Remember, you can be as sexually ecstatic as you choose to be!

Believe it or not, there's an awe-inspiring natural psychological law that basically says you are what you think about. Whether positive or negative, we become what we concentrate and focus on most of the time. This is a powerful concept, yet relatively easy to do. Systematic purposeful concentration leads to successful actualization of any goal. So if we do this on a habitual basis, those thoughts become an integral part of our lives. Why not think about *spirited sex*? Not only ponder it, but also vocalize, write, act, and dream about it.

I only have one more word of advice. Actually, it's two sentences. A Zen Buddhist might suggest the same thought-provoking counsel:

Absorb this book, then forget what you've read while making love! Let your heart and soul be your guide!

Homework Assignment

Try these during the next thirty days. You'll be glad you did! (I'm interested in your results. Please write me: Janalee Beck, c/o LifeQuest, P.O. Box 25786, Tempe, AZ 85285–5786.)

Take a hot, leisurely bath (while the kids are gone or asleep) and surround the tub with as many candles as you desire. Listening to music is optional.

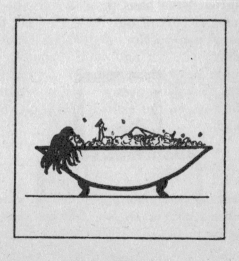

Relaxation is mandatory. You may use a wash-cloth or just soap on your hands, and notice how your body feels when you wash it. Try it rough or tender, slow or fast, hard or soft. Each and every sensation provides stimulation.

Watch a sensual (erotic) movie with or without your partner. Recommendations include: *Body Heat; The Unbearable Lightness of Being; Wife-mistress; Sex, Lies, and Videotape;* and *9½ Weeks.*

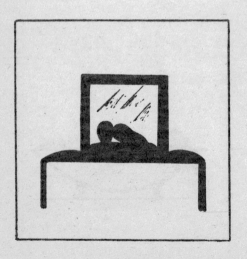

Any movie that makes you feel sensual would be a good choice. Personally, I like the old-fashioned black-and-white classics!

Engage in "phone foreplay." Call your partner at odd, unsuspecting times. Leave a message on his answering machine. This may INSPIRE him. Then again, don't expect too much. If nothing happens, just try again another time. He'll love it!

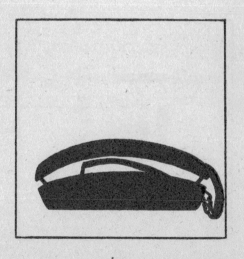

For example: "Hi, sweetheart, I was just thinking about you and got horny as heck. If I had a chance right this minute I'd..." (*Well, you get the idea!*)